CONFESSIONS OF A
CERTIFIED
PERSONAL
TRAINER

CONFESSIONS OF A
CERTIFIED
PERSONAL
TRAINER

Volume I
The Fitness Revolution
Educating you on the
right way to exercise

ROBERT LINKUL

MS NSCA-CPT D* CSCS D*

Printed in the United States of America.

ISBN: 978-1-4269-7267-6 (sc)
ISBN: 978-1-4269-7268-3 (e)

Trafford rev. 06/16/2011

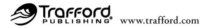 www.trafford.com

North America & International
toll-free: 1 888 232 4444 (USA & Canada)
phone: 250 383 6864 ♦ fax: 812 355 4082

Confessions of a Certified Personal Trainer
Educating You on the Right Way to Exercise

Volume I: Welcome to the Fitness Revolution
By Robert Linkul MS CSCS D*

Introduction

My name is Robert Linkul, and I am a Certified Personal Trainer with the National Strength and Conditioning Association (NSCA). I am the NSCA's Northern California State Director, the "Career Builder" columnist for Personal Fitness Professional (PFP) Magazine's website, and the Head Personal Trainer at Arden Hills Resort Club and Spa in Sacramento, California. I earned my first personal training certification in 1999. I later received my Bachelors degree in Kinesiology from California State University at Sacramento in 2005, and became a certified strength and conditioning specialist in 2007. In 2008, I earned my Masters degree in Personal Training from the United States Sports Academy.

Since I began my education in physical fitness over twelve years ago, I have committed myself to learning as much as possible about the personal training business, and I would like to share some of this knowledge with you. This book originated from a fitness-based newsletter (which you can sign up for by emailing me at robertlinkul@ gmail.com or "friend" me at www.facebook.com/robert.linkul) as well as some research papers and recent publications.

From this book, I hope you find inspiration. I have poured into it my passion for the personal training business and the fitness industry. Thank you for purchasing my book, and I hope you enjoy it.

Thank you

I would like to say thank you to my wife, Keagan, for having patience with me over the last year of our lives. I have spent many hours working on this project, and her continued support encouraged me to put into it everything I had. Thank you, Honey!

Thank you to my parents, Richard and Tina, for supporting every single thing I do. Their constant love and support is there whenever I need it, and I call on them often to receive it. Thank you both for raising me, for loving me, and for being proud of me. I love you both very much!

Thank you to my sister Amanda and her husband Rene for their spiritual influences. I am very passionate about being surrounded by positive people with good energy and I couldn't find two more positive people to be in my life. I love you both. Thank you for your guidance.

Lastly, thank you to the NSCA, to PFP magazine and to Arden Hills Resort Club and Spa for the opportunities they have offered me. I hope I make you all proud. Again, thank you.

What Is the Fitness Revolution?

Over the last 12 years of my career I have developed a different perspective on typical thinking styles pertaining to fitness, personal training and program design. I wanted to make sure I was teaching and implementing the absolute best ways to train to my clients, so, I decided to become a continued education junky. Since 1999, I have attended over 30 seminars, conferences, clinics, camps and symposiums. I have read as many books as I could get my hands on; I have read research papers, strength and conditioning journals and self-studies. All of this information has lead to a new way of thinking about exercise and a more non-traditional style of training.

As a society, we are often fed incorrect information and presented with unhealthy life style images to aspire toward. We are taught that being fat makes you an "ugly person," that women have to be sickly thin to be considered "sexy," and that a six-pack is the only way to have a "strong core," along with many other misleading stereotypes. The

Fitness Revolution is a new way of thinking and an improved way of training. This thought process utilizes education and passion to fuel the energy needed to achieve the fitness related goals that each and every one of us has.

Fitness should be fun, it should be something we look forward to and it shouldn't hurt our bodies in any way (other than being sore). We are unique people trying to achieve something great, whatever our fitness goals may be. The Fitness Revolution is your guide to assure you that you are training correctly. Disband the myths, and learn the right way to exercise. Once you begin this journey, please make sure you remain focused and, as I like to say, "Stay the course".

This book is called "Confessions of a Certified Personal Trainer," meaning that all of the information in this book is put together from years of reading research papers, journals and books. I have listed many of them below for you to reference. I often refer to "recent studies" in this book and those studies come form this list. These are my confessions, not a research paper and I want this book to read like you are having a conversation with me. This is why I often do not cite my work. Enjoy, and if you have any questions please do not hesitate to email me.

robertlinkul@gmail.com

Books Referenced:

- **The New Rules of Lifting for Women**
    - By Lou Schuler, Cassandra Forsythe and Alwyn Cosgrove (2007)

- **The New Rules of Lifting: Six Basic Moves for Maximum Muscle**
    - By Lou Schuler and Alwyn Cosgrove (2006)

- **The New Rules of Lifting for Abs**
    - By Lou Schuler and Alwyn Cosgrove (2010)

- **The Total Body Breakthrough**
  - By Multiple Authors (2010)

- **The Complete Guide to Kettle Bell Lifting**
  - By Steve Cotter (2009)

- **The Female Body Breakthrough**
  - By Rachel Cosgrove (2009)

- **The Impact Body Plan**
  - By Todd Durkin, Adam Bornstein and Mike Zimmerman (2010)

- **Fifty Five Business Strategies for Success**
  - By Rachel and Alwyn Cosgrove (2009)

- **Movement: Functional Movement Systems**
  - Gray Cook (2010)

- **Advances in Functional Training**
  - By Michael Boyle (2010)

- **The Body Fat Solution**
  - By Tom Venuto (2009)

- **Maximum Strength**
  - By Eric Cressey and Matt Fitzgerald (2008)

- **NSCA's Strength and Conditioning Journals**
  - December 2006 to April 2011

- **Strength Training: National Strength & Conditioning Association**
  - Edited by Lee E. Brown (2007)

It Begins: The Fitness Revolution

We have all seen "Mr. Gimmick" in the weight room. You know, the guy who is doing bicep curls while standing on one bare foot in the middle of a Bosu ball, his eyes closed while chanting his mantra. Beware of "Mr. Gimmick", as he may injure others around him in addition to himself while attempting his next trick… I mean exercise. What is the point of the new "Gimmick" exercise equipment? I wish I had an answer for you. The best I can come up with is that I think people simply get bored. To keep things interesting, trainers create these "new" pieces of equipment that are "going to change the fitness industry forever." I have seen weighted clubs, bowling pins, thigh masters, inner-tubes, parachute harnesses, giant medicine balls, wheels with handles on them, ropes to walk on, suspension bungees to bounce from, and more. All of these "gimmick" pieces of equipment are knock-offs of other, more traditional, pieces of equipment but they have a new spin on them. In reality, they are not going to change much at all, because they are gimmicks. The greatest piece of fitness equipment has already been created. It's called a "barbell."

The traditional exercises have been around forever because they work. It is very difficult in this day and age to create a new exercise or to invent a piece of exercise equipment. Biomechanically speaking, we have reached our potential in regards to fitness machines and creating the best angle of pull or push. The dumbbell, barbell and kettlebell have been around forever because they work (check out Steve Cotters 'The Complete Guide to Kettel Bell Lifting" This is all you really need. Maybe add a pair of gymnastics rings and a medicine ball, but other than that, I'm good to go.

Instead of creating some new piece of equipment, I used to select just one piece of already existing equipment and would try to train each of my clients with it. This forced me to be creative. We would do an entire workout, working our entire bodies with just one dumbbell or one medicine ball. Designing workouts with a goal of working every muscle in the body really tested my creativity. In the long run, this helped me create a large variety of exercises that keeps my workouts fresh, challenging, and innovative.

Please, do not fall into the "gimmick" trap. Do not buy those goofy machines, apparatuses and contraptions. There is no piece of machinery or exercise program in the entire world that you can perform for "six minutes a day" and get the body you have always dreamed of (trust me, if there was, I would have found it by now). We all know - it takes hard work.

There comes a time in each person's life when he or she has finally had enough, and wants to make the effort to lead a healthier life by improving eating habits and increasing physical activity. This moment has come to me many times. In turn, many times I have dramatically changed my body either by leaning out or bulking up. I hope this moment in life happens to you if you have not already experienced it. When you make the choice to change your body and improve the quality of your health, you will feel proud. You will feel good all day long. You will no longer need coffee to wake you up mid-day because your endorphins from your workout at lunch time will do it for you. You will sleep better at night, you will have a better sex drive, and you will become more energetic during the day and feel vibrant once again.

I have recently experienced this feeling. I have had some health issues in the past including a ruptured disc in my back in 2008 (L5-S1), lung cancer in 2009 (Carcinoid tumor) and thyroiditis in 2010 (Hashimoto's disease). As I began to heal following these setbacks, I have made changes to my eating and exercise habits, and noticed a change almost immediately. I sleep and feel so much better than I did in the past. I owe it all to my wife. She encouraged me and motivated me to change the way I live my life - what kind of food I ate, what type of work I committed to, and how often I exercised. I owe this dramatic change in my life to her and I couldn't be more appreciative. I can only hope, for those of you who may be lost out there, that you find your way.

I call this the "fitness revolution." I aim to change the way people view, think about and experience fitness. I hope these newsletters help you to change the way you think about your personal fitness goals and influence you to take your health into your own hands and make a change for the better. Please feel free to email or call me anytime, as this is my passion in life. I will be happy to discuss or assist you in any way. Let your "fitness revolution" begin for you today! Make a change. You deserve it!

Finding My Perfect Body

Since 1999 when I entered the personal training business, I have had clients ask me about helping them transform their bodies into a different body type as their fitness goal. Some want look like "super models". Some want to pump up like "Arnold". Others want the thin, lithe "runner's body". It is hard for me as the professional to answer them by saying that we are all genetically created to have a certain type of body frame from birth. Our genetics dictate which body type each of us will grow into if trained correctly.

Generally speaking, each of us fits into one of three body types: endomorph, ectomorph, and mesomorph. There is some overlap between these forms and varieties do exist, but, generally speaking, most of us fit into one of these categories.

Endomorphs have a great ability to put on muscle and have a hard time losing fat; built for lifting, not so much for running. They tend to be more broad in the shoulder and hips and are rather large (not fat) in stature. Ectomorphs are exactly the opposite. They struggle to put on muscle and can lose fat in a blink of an eye. They are generally good at completing long, slow distances, but are not extremely strong. They tend to be long and lean (not skinny) in stature. Mesomorphs are right in the middle. They can put on some size and lose some fat and tend to be centered when it comes to size and stature.

One is not better than the others. However, we need to discover which category you fall into and next prescribe an appropriate sport or activity. For example, an endomorph may not be the best candidate for running a marathon, and an ectomorph would have a lot of trouble trying to back squat their body weight.

Of course, each of these body types has its own exceptions, based on muscle fibers and such. These are generalizations and are by no means permanent diagnoses. I personally know some endomorphs who are exceptional runners based on having such a high type I muscle fiber count.

If you would like to train for a culminating event (an athletic event on a set date for which you can set personal goals) but do not know which event your body type would be most appropriate for, please email me and we can schedule an appointment to discuss it. There are many options to choose from. Having a goal to work toward makes training much more valuable. The specific event you choose gives you a reason to work just a little bit harder each day. Additionally, it helps prevent you from missing a workout because you're "just not feeling it today."

Not all of us are genetically designed to have the runner's body or to look like Arnold. But this doesn't mean we can't try our best to achieve the look we want. We simply need an appropriate game plan and a designed program to help us achieve that goal. Don't feel lost. There is an answer out there for us; we just need to find it.

Cardio Queens

Studies conducted over the past fifteen years or so suggest that long term cardiovascular exercise (20+ minutes) at the same level for the same amount of time day in and day out will not help to reduce body fat. Let me say that again: doing the treadmill every morning on a 4% incline at 3 miles per hour for 30 minutes is not helping you change your body composition. Of course it has its benefits for individuals who are rehabilitating an injury or something of that nature. However, if you are a fully functioning individual and you are maintaining this daily exercise routine, you are what we call a "Cardio Queen."

Studies also show that performing weight training interval workout routines two or three days a week for 30 minutes will dramatically change the composition of your body if you follow a proper nutrition program and work as hard as you can during your workouts. In fact, you will burn NINE times more FAT then the "Cardio Queen" who performs 45 minutes of constant cardio FIVE times a week.

To recap, lifting weights at a high interval rate three days a week for 30 minutes will burn NINE times more FAT then running/walking on a treadmill/elliptical/stair stepper/Etc. for five days a week for 45 minutes. The fact is, this is the best way for you to transform your body into what you want it to be.

My favorite book on the market right now discusses this same idea (I don't get a kick down if you buy the book - if I did you would have heard about it a long time ago ☺). *The Female Body Breakthrough* by Rachel Cosgrove changed the way I train my clients to this day. Although it is directed at women, the message pertains to men as well: lift weights to change your body. Because my clients are 90 percent women, I thought it would be a great book to read. You should have seen me in line waiting to buy my copy and have it signed with 60 other females (I was the only male in sight). Needless to say, she was shocked to see me and asked, "Are you lost?"

Regardless of whether it is geared toward men or women, the take home message is the same for everyone. Change up your routine daily, and work weights into your workout routine. The same consistent lack of challenge will continue to maintain an unchanged you. You need a new and improved "you". Start by mixing it up with the weights. Remember, the weight room is not a scary place for women. My weight room is overrun by women for eight hours every day. Get in there and lift, ladies! You won't get big and bulky! You will only get stronger and leaner and obtain great looking bodies!

We Must Improve Our Bust!

I'm not old enough know from where or when the saying "We must improve our bust" came from. However, I remember several teenage girls using a Thigh Master type of machine on their upper body with the idea that if they made their chest muscles stronger, their breasts would grow larger. Try as they might, these girls never achieved their desired results using this method. This is a great example of the exercise myth regarding "site specific reduction" or, in this case, enhancement.

I'm sorry to say there is no such thing as "site specific reduction". By that, I mean that you cannot burn away fat from one specific location on your body by performing an exercise on that area. Yes, I know ladies, you have been doing those hips and buns exercises for years. Sorry, it hasn't been working for you! The one thing it has been doing is making the muscles in that area stronger. The secret to fat loss (which is no secret at all) is exercise and diet. Period.

The concept of site specific reduction reminds me of a story one of my clients told me about her mother. One day, she was driving with the car window down and her arm out the window. She kept hearing a "thump thump thump" noise, and eventually pulled over to check if her tire was flat. She got back in her car after finding every tire intact and continued to drive. Once she regained speed, the noise returned. It turned out that it was her "arm flab" blowing in the wind and hitting the side of the car door, in turn making the noise.

Everyone has their trouble areas (myself included), and we all want to make them go away or look better. The way to succeed in doing so is to have a program designed for you that will both increase your overall strength and cardiovascular endurance at the same time. Include a healthy diet and stay consistent and you WILL see results over time.

Bringing the discussion back to the "we must improve our bust" line - yes, it is possible to increase the size of a specific body part by working the muscles underneath the area in question. A study was performed which measured a group of women's chest circumferences before and after a chest dominant workout. The results showed a half inch increase in size following the workout. This is a result of something called the "pump", which occurs when a large amount of blood is pushed into a muscle during and following excessive use. Some of you may have felt this and know that always feels good. If you can continue to produce this "pump" time and time again, the muscles being worked will begin to grow stronger and thus increase in size.

Ladies, don't freak out. You are not going to go up a cup size. Muscles are like plants; if you water them they will grow, but only as big as they are intended to grow. With proper training, your muscles will get stronger, not "too bulky." My message for today - don't be afraid to be strong! Embrace your strength. It will only make you better.

CPT Business: First Impressions, Lasting Relationships
(Published on PFP Website "Career Builder" Column 2011 – May)

A good first impression is vital to the success of a Certified Personal Training business. We give our first impressions through personal assessments, which provide us with the opportunity to establish professional and personal connections with potential clients. Usually, a connection will lead to a client scheduling his or her first session. From there, he or she can potentially become a "lifer." If a successful connection is not made, we as professionals should make every effort to match the respective client with a trainer who's strengths are more compatible with the client's needs with the hope that a successful relationship will be developed. Regardless, this first impression lays the foundation to build a successful business.

In the personal training business, it is extremely important that we offer each client an initial assessment. During these assessments, we get to interact with potential clients to see if we will enjoy working with them. Sometimes it is hard to tell if you and your potential client are going to gel. In this case, offer them a free workout session. This gives both of you another opportunity to see if the relationship is going to work. It's similar to dating; you might have to meet up for coffee once or twice before you decide to ask them out to dinner and a movie.

In the beginning of my personal training career, I would work with any client I came across just to make a living. As I quickly learned, it is more important to enjoy the company of the individual I work with than to attempt to establish a connection that is not meant to be. This makes for a much more enjoyable individual session, and improves my energy level throughout the day.

The truth is every personal trainer has had a client he or she does not enjoy training. For a while, I had a client during the last time slot in my Tuesday schedule that I could not stand. Every Tuesday, I spent the entire day dreading this session. But, I forced myself to train her so I could make some money. Over time, I began to hate working on Tuesdays entirely. My energy was different starting on Tuesday mornings and, as each hour drew my hated client nearer, my mood grew worse. My other clients began to sense this negative attitude and grew irritated with me. Next thing I knew, my business was no longer improving, and I even became known as "the grumpy trainer".

The energy we emit during each and every physical training session in turn feeds our client's energy level. My mentor once told me that we are not allowed to have "bad days" because we are, in many cases, the best part of our clients' days. They come to us because they need encouragement, and are looking for someone to lead them in the right direction. Many of our clients sit at desks all day long staring at computer screens. We are their saving grace, and therefore need to provide them with an enthusiastic and positive workout experience. This will leave each of them feeling better, and cause them to look forward to their next training session.

Obviously, it is important to make a living. However, it cannot be at the cost of ruining the quality of the product we provide. If you feel during your initial assessment that the relationship is not going to work, refer that client to another trainer. Yes, you will be losing money at that moment. However, you also benefit because it will not ruin the quality of your product in the long run. Only train the clients that with whom you feel a positive connection. Although it may take some extra time and effort, you will eventually establish a full schedule of clients that you look forward to and thoroughly enjoy training. Surrounding yourself with positive people will bring the best out of you and will in turn lead to referrals from your pleased clients.

In the beginning, it may feel odd to turn away potential business opportunities. If you trust yourself to get a good sense of the people you meet, then you can create a following of individuals that you enjoy getting to know and truly look forward to working with each and every hour. From there, a trainer can reach his "dream job" because he gets to work only with the individuals he enjoys. Do not be afraid to assess and train a client for free to make certain your relationship is going to be successful. It will pay off in the long run.

Nothing Is Over

You will not find a bigger John J. Rambo fan (*First Blood, First Blood Part II, Part III, Rambo*) than me. I grew up wanting to be just like Sylvester Stallone. I wanted muscles, but didn't want to be *too* big. Those of you who know me know I'm also a huge Arnold Schwarzenegger fan. However, even at age ten I knew I had a better chance of looking like Rambo then I did the Terminator.

Anyway, in the first Rambo movie, Stallone became famous for his line, "Nothing is over!" This got me thinking. I have heard so many of my clients say that they've tried to diet and it didn't work, or that they tried working out and didn't like it. Not everyone likes watching "The Bachelor" (I do!) and not everyone enjoys "Glee" (I don't!). However, most people find and stick with television shows they enjoy. The same goes for healthy eating and exercise. You need to find exercise and eating habits that *you* like, because then you are certainly more likely to keep them up. Continue to try new workout routines and experimenting with different dietary plans. Eventually, you will find one that both fits your needs and is enjoyable. For those of you out there who say, "I hate all exercise and I want to eat what I eat and that's just the way it is. It's over", my words to you are, "NOTHING IS OVER!"

If you struggle with diet and working out, you need to find foods and exercises you can manage and enjoy. If you have a bad back, start riding a recumbent bike. If you have achy joints, start swimming. If your shoulders hurt reaching straight up over head, try taking up golf (it does wonders for flexibility!). Some of us who have been competitive athletes may think that life has passed us by following aging or injury. Stop talking about the "Glory Days" and try something new. You need to find something you can be passionate about. You should enjoy your physical activity and YES, there is an activity out there for everyone! You just need to find it.

My message is this. I know I'm no Stallone or Schwarzenegger, and I will never be because of my back (my ruptured disc doesn't allow me to squat or dead lift heavy anymore). Regardless, I have found a form of exercise that makes me feel good, that I enjoy, that I look forward to and that is producing results. Steve Cotter's kettle bell training has literally changed the way I exercise. Kettle bell training has helped improve my lower back issues, my flexibility and increased my full body strength.

I believe deep in my heart that there is something like this out there for you. Find something you can be excited about. Without passion, we have nothing to live for. If it's your kids you feel passion for, get out and play sports with them. If it's your spouse, go out on a walk or bike ride together. Whatever you do, please seek your passion and start to change the quality of your life today. Remember Rambo. "Nothing is over."

Just Makin' 'Em Sweat

The majority of personal trainers I have met since joining the business maintains that clients do not care why they are doing the exercises their trainer asks them to perform. When I question them on this topic, I usually get a response like, "my clients just want to sweat." Hearing a professional say something like this physically makes me ill. If you are currently training with a trainer and you do not care why you are performing the exercises you are performing, I urge you to reinvest in your body and learn about what you are doing.

I think of myself as an educator as well as a trainer. I have mentored and am currently mentoring other trainers to gain what I call, "Jerry McGuire Syndrome." Jerry McGuire Syndrome encourages the trainer to look at his or her clients as actual people who have feelings rather than just as paychecks. It also emphasizes learning to be empathetic, compassionate, honest, and, when need be, stern when conducting a personal training session. Most of all, I urge them to care about what they are teaching their clients.

Let me give you an example demonstrating the importance of a trainer's investment in what he instructs. When returning from my lunch break a few years back, I found a coworker instructing a woman on how to perform pull-ups. He had a 65 year-old woman, 30 pounds overweight, standing on the front three inches of a chair (on her tip toes) with a 110-pound resistant band around her feet (we use these by tying them to the pull up bar and then hooking the other end around the clients feet to give them assistance pulling up). Her fingertips were just barely around the bar. To top it all off, he was not spotting the client or holding the chair. His focus was on a younger girl in the room working out instead of focusing on his client.

Images of this woman losing her grip and falling backwards as the band sprung upward flipping her 180 degrees (head first toward the floor) and hitting her head on the chair below flashed through my mind. There are so many issues with this situation, but I'll just pick out three. Firstly, she is 30 pounds overweight and pull-ups are not a realistic goal at that point. She should be on a pull down machine to develop some of the basic strength requirements needed to perform a chin up.

Second of all, standing on a chair is, for anyone let alone a 65-year-old woman, a dangerous position. She should be on the floor or on a plyometric or step up box to help her reach the bar more safely. Lastly, she can hardly reach the bar. Even my strongest clients have trouble performing a pull up from the "dead hang" position.

It is dangerous, it's malpractice, and it is performed every day in gyms across the country. My message to other trainers is this: you owe it to yourself to be better than that. Have some passion about what you do and understand that having respect for and teaching your client the importance of safe exercising is a large part of the job. Otherwise, get out of this business and find what you are passionate about. Try to help your clients to achieve something meaningful and safe rather than "just makin' 'em sweat."

My message to the client: don't ever be afraid to ask your trainer why you are performing a certain exercise. If they can't give you an answer, or they answer with "because it's hard", you need to find someone else with whom to work. Find a trainer who is going to take you somewhere, and who will help you achieve your goal. If you have been with the same trainer for years and nothing has changed, I hate to say it, but IT'S NOT WORKING! Find someone else.

I believe in being as professional as possible with every one of my clients. I want them to leave every session thinking that they learned something, that they are moving toward achieving their personal fitness goal and that it was worth their money. If I can look myself in the mirror every morning and say "I'm passionate and I'm going to make a difference in someone else's life today" and mean it, I know that I am in the right profession.

Is it Hot in Here or Is It Just Me?

Earlier in 2010, I was diagnosed with Thyroiditis (also known as Hashimoto disease) which caused my thyroid to continually grow larger. Because of this, I had my thyroid removed, which in turn caused my hormone levels to drop and become uneven. Because of my low and uneven hormone levels, I now experience hot flashes on a daily basis. I often joke with my mother that I now know what she felt when she went through menopause, but this is hardly a joking matter for most women. Every woman will experience warning signs and go through menopause at some point in her aging process. Menopause can also be brought on following a surgery, such as a hysterectomy, and can often lead to extreme symptoms.

I am far from an expert when it comes to this topic. However, I do train many women who are near to or are currently experiencing menopause. Because of my frequent interaction with female clients, I decided to educate myself on the topic. I signed up for a six week class called "Training the Aging Women", which taught me to recognize the warning signs and make the appropriate changes to my program design and nutritional suggestions to make my client(s) more comfortable.

Heading the list of menopause symptoms is my favorite, hot flashes, followed by mood swings, depression, and cold sweats. Because of the lack of or low amounts of estrogen and progesterone in the body, the naturally occurring monthly cycle stops. This changes what the body has been used to for the last 40 to 60 years, and in turn causes major hormonal changes. A diet high in fresh vegetables, fruit, whole grains, and beans and low in red meat and saturated fat can bring relief from many of these symptoms.

A consistent exercise routine should accompany a clean diet. Exercise will boost mental wellbeing and increase bone density, strengthen muscles, improve digestion, and increase circulation. Women who exercise reported that their health was "better" or "much better" when compared to those who did not exercise during menopause. This study also reported that physical activity helped them to maintain an appropriate body composition for their age, height and weight.

Exercise has proven to make the transition into menopause much easier for the average female. Maintaining a consistent exercise routine as well as a healthy and well balanced diet can make the menopause side effects much more comfortable. If you or someone you know is experiencing all or some of these symptoms, I advise you to go see your doctor prior to beginning any exercise routine. Exercise can improve your quality of life before, during and after menopause. Don't wait. Get active today.

It's All in the Hips

One of my favorite movies is based on a former "fight-first" hot headed hockey player with a wicked-bad slap shot named Happy Gilmore. Skating, an essential ability in ice hockey, is not one of his strongest points, and his lacking skills eventually get him cut from the team. His world falls around him as his dreams go up in smoke. In turn, however, he accidentally discovers that his wicked-bad slap shot gives him a great advantage when hitting a golf ball. His only problem? Putting. He struggles because he has no control of his hips. To help him, he finds a coach named "Chapps," who, after having his hand bitten off by an alligator, became a professional golfer. I know, I know, it sounds stupid, but I swear I have a point coming up soon, so bare with me.

A simple physical movement like putting in golf has so many technical points that it is hard to put them all together to perform the act perfectly. The body weight squat (back squat, front squat, sumo squat, over-head squat, etc.) is very similar. Like putting, the secret to a good squat is "all in the hips". I use a term called "hip displacement" to describe the correct processes of squatting. Many individuals I work with at first simply bend their knees until they think they are low enough and then stand up. The more the knee bends and displaces forward beyond the toes, the more unnecessary pressure is placed on the patella (patellar tendon and ligament). The average patella is about 2"x2"x1" inches in size. If an average sized person is 5' 8" tall and weighs 170 pounds, the pressure placed on this tiny little bone, ligament and tendon is massive and will cause it to only last so long.

When performed correctly, with "hip displacement," all the pressure is applied to the larger muscles of the legs and primarily the gluteus muscles (the butt). The gluteus muscles are thick, dense and massive. Their primary job (other than to look good) is to extend the leg. The gluteus, 8"x4"x2" (on average), is a much more efficient muscle on which to place all of the pressure otherwise being placed on the patella. Now that we know which area is best to use, how do we use it?

"Hip displacement" starts from the standing position. Place your feet slightly wider then shoulder width with your toes slightly out to the sides. Without bending the knees, stick out your rear as far as possible while keeping your chest (sternum) up and the weight of the body on the heels. Once the rear is out as far as possible, begin to bend the knees in place (keep them from moving forward) until the crease of the hips is parallel with the knee joint. This is a hard action to master. I have been working with clients for over ten years, and many still need reminding on how to do it correctly. It helps to place yourself next to a mirror and watch the knee joint as you perform your movement. It also helps to have someone kneel next to you and hold the knee joint in place while you try to squat correctly.

Squatting is a movement that each of us performs multiple times a day. Like an electrical wire, your knees will last a while but will eventually wear out and fail if you don't take care of them. When getting up from your chair at work, sitting down on the couch at home, or when exercising, remember coach Chapps holding Happy's hands and whispering, "It's all in the hips, Baby".

Because I Can Feel It

I am often asked, "Why don't we do more abdominal work during our training session?" I consistently answer that question with, "Everything we do is abdominal work." If you have worked with me before, you know that I have adopted the training concept of no 'Old School' abdominal exercises (sit ups, crunches, medicine ball sit ups, etc.) I wasn't always this way. When I first started training clients, I had everyone do these exercises at the end of our workout routine just as would every other trainer in America. I continued with this training philosophy until I injured myself in 2008. I ruptured a disc in my lumbar due to years of incorrect squatting technique and from millions of repetitions of 'Old School' abdominal exercises.

You may have heard this saying, "Those who can no longer do, teach." I am a really good example of that saying. As I began to rehabilitate myself, I discovered how much those 'Old School' abdominal exercises hurt me. My doctors said I had to get my core stronger, and this was the only way I knew how. I needed to feel my abdominals burning. If it burned, then I knew it was working. After two weeks of attempting to rehabilitate myself in this manner I realized that I was making my injury worse. I decided to take a step back and look at my situation anatomically.

Vertebra stack on top of each other similarly to the way large Lego blocks stack together. In between these Lego pieces are vertebra discs. The disc is similar to a very solid jelly donut. If there is too much weight placed on the vertebra above the disc the jelly will squirt out the side. This is what happened to me. While in the supine position (lying on my back face up) and rolling my chest toward my pelvis I was in fact creating an inverted spinal column. This meant that I was forcing the spine in the exact opposite direction it wants to go. Doing this caused my pelvis to tilt upward as well as make the pain in my back twice as bad. It was then that I realized that these 'Old School' training habits where not good for me at all, and I need to make a change.

I found that my most pain free positions were standing perfectly straight or lying perfectly flat. Either way, my spine was where it should be, straightened out rather than hunched over. Perfect posture became my personal practice. Because of my experiences rehabilitating from this injury, I now teach perfect posture during every exercise my clients perform. Think about your body in the plank position (a push up position on your forearms instead of your hands). If turned up right that would be a standing position, so I applied my perfect posture rule to it: hips out and chest up. Back squats became hips out chest up, push-ups became hips out chest up, bent over rows became hips up chest out... you get the idea. I applied this rule to everything I did, and this made my core muscles very strong again.

The perfect posture position is the strongest core position that you can have. If there is any deviation in this position (hunching of the shoulders, dropping of the hips, rounding of the butt, etc.), then the core shows its signs of weakness. When I tell my clients that we are constantly doing core work, it is because we are always in that perfectly postured position. The next workout you do, actually, the next time you do *anything*, think about having your hips slightly out and your chest pointing upwards. Try sitting at your desk this way for three minutes, and see how tired your core muscles become. It can be exhausting.

I practice what I preach, and I hope that you will too. Attempting to bring the chest toward the pelvis (sit ups) may give you the sensation that you are working those muscles more effectively when, in actuality, you are harming them. Do not perform an exercise just so you can "feel it." Perform exercises with a purpose. If you have any questions on this topic, please feel free to email me. I know this is a popular topic; I could write I lot more on it. However, I don't want to bore you all. Keep that posture perfect for every movement that you perform and your core will be at its strongest. I guarantee it! Stay the course and thank you for joining the fitness revolution.

Hard Times Bring Hard Decisions

As our economy has taken a turn for the worse, many have been forced to cut multiple expenses from their budgets. These cut expenses unfortunately frequently include gym memberships. In a time where mental and physical health is taxed by heavy stress, the last thing people should do is cut exercise out of their life. Many commit to working out at home, or going jogging with a friend. After a few weeks, that commitment is forgotten as other home duties take priority.

Exercise has many effects that are vital for mental and physical health, and in turn greatly reduce stress levels. Exercising releases hormones that increase quality of sleep, focusing and thinking abilities, energy levels, sex life, and more. Improvements in all of these areas assist in reducing stress levels and improve one's quality of life. Exercise reduces risk of disease throughout the human body, improves posture, increases flexibility, and reduces the risk of injury. The benefits of exercising could dramatically improve the quality of life of the stressed individual. Because of this, it is suggested that we, as a society, spend more time exercising.

Our country's obesity levels are higher than ever before, and are also higher than those of any other country in the world. The same goes for childhood obesity. The lifestyle consisting of fast and easily accessible food is literally destroying our bodies and, in turn, is destroying our society. Health and fitness should be the highest priorities on the list. Without our health, what do we have?

Cutting the funds for health and fitness out of a budget is an easy decision to make because they may seem like accessories rather than staples. However, the costs of not exercising can be catastrophic (like death!). Taking small steps toward changing your diet and fitness level is a great way to slowly change the ill effects of stress and poor health. It takes a long period of time, in some cases, years, to deplete the health of the human body. Fortunately, years of poor diet and lack of exercise can be fixed rather quickly. It takes a committed individual and a strong support system, but can be done.

Personal trainers are educated and experienced in working with people who fit the description of unhealthy. Making the financial and emotional commitment to work with a certified fitness professional is the best way to make a dramatic change.

These are hard times, and eating poorly and not exercising only makes them harder. The decision to change ourselves both mentally and physically is up to us. Take a step in the right direction and schedule a session with a certified fitness professional to make a life style change for the better.

Just Gonna Go for a Run

I have heard almost every excuse out there as to why a client can't make it to a workout. My problem is not with the excuse, but rather with one particular sentence that follows the excuse. One of my favorite clients text messaged me one morning and said that she isn't going to be able to make our scheduled weight training session because of "enter excuse here."

She then follows the excuse with, "I'm just gonna go for a run" when her schedule allows for it. All you runners out there please don't take this the wrong way. Running is not weight training. Yes, running can be a great workout or part of a great workout routine, but the benefits of weight training are far and above when compared to running. Let's take a look at both of these areas of exercise and break down their components.

Running works the cardiovascular system extremely well, and does provide an increase to muscular endurance by contracting the same muscles over and over again for a long period of time. Running is also a plyometric activity. Plyometric is defined as an explosive movement that puts the body into flight. In this case, every stride taken produces a small "flight" stage where both feet are not on the ground.

The average mile consists of 1,500 strides. The average runner produces two and a half times their body weight in pressure per stride when running. For example, a man who weighs 200 pounds takes one stride in a running motion and places 500 pounds of pressure on that one foot. The next step, 500 pounds, the next, 500 pounds and so on. After a mile, this man has placed over 750,000 pounds of pressure on his joints.

My point is this: when beginners say, "I'm going to get in shape starting tomorrow by going for a run", they are about to perform one of the worst possible things to their body at that point. Running is a physical activity requiring proper technique that needs to be developed over time. There are coaches who make very good livings by strictly teaching people proper running mechanics.

Without proper progression and technique, the body will eventually be devastated by so much impact. Posture will break down, bone density will begin to decrease or splint, and muscle mass will begin to shrink (atrophy) if weight training is not included in a person's exercising schedule. Weight training increases bone density, muscle mass (hypertrophy), and core strength, all without the heavy pounding on the joints.

A correct weight training program called High Intensity Training (HIT) can increase cardiovascular endurance and muscular endurance just as well as running can without the pounding of the joints. I successfully trained a young lady to qualify for the Boston marathon in 2010 from running twice a week and HIT three to four times a week. Her injuries were dramatically decreased from her past marathon training, which included running four to five days a week and hardly any weight training.

My message is this: if you are going to run, you need to train for the sport of running. You can't just go out and run like Michael Johnson; it takes years of practice and proper training (and a pair of gold Nike shoes). If your goal is to get into good all around physical shape, I suggest you start your new routine in the weight room. Once your body is stronger and can handle some of the pounding that running produces, you can start adding in a day or two of short runs. Remember, running is a high impact activity and you will need time to recover from it. Seek the advice and guidance of a professional if need be.

I am not an "anti-running" type of guy. I'm an "anti-running when your body is not strong enough to handle running" type of guy.

Cause Baby It's Cold Outside

When the fall season arrives, I am in heaven. I love the change in colors as well as the drop in the temperature. I enjoy the cooler weather, and love being outdoors in it. Exercising outside becomes more enjoyable. It takes a minute or two for my body to warm up but, before I know it, I'm stripping down the layers to cool off a bit. Then comes winter, when warming up becomes a little harder and more important than before. Warming up for exercise outdoors during the blazing heat of the summer seems to take mere seconds compared to the lengthy time spent warming up in winter. Here are some tips for the next time you go out to exercise in the cold.

Always dress in layers. Thinner layers insulate the heat on your body much better than one or two big thick jackets or sweatshirts. As your body begins to warm up, a layer can be taken off every few minutes until you find a comfort level. If, for example, the pace of your run decreases or the wind begins to pick up, you can add another layer to make up the difference. On a pure comfort note, it's much easier, based on size, to deal with layers (tie it around your waste or pack it into a bag) than it is to deal with a down jacket.

When you think you are warmed up, warm up a little more. There are times when your body will be feeling warm based on your metabolism or, if you are a female, on certain times of the month. Don't mistake this hot or warm sensation for your muscles being warmed up. It is always better to do a little too much warming up than not enough. A pulled or torn muscle can keep you on the shelf for weeks, or even months. Putting in a little extra energy prior to your exercise routine to ensure your safety is worth it. A note for competitors: this does not apply to pre-competition warm ups. You want to save as much energy as possible for the competition. Practice warming yourself up days before the event at the same time of day during which you will be competing so you know exactly how much time it takes for you to feel ready. On competition day, every bit of energy counts.

In extreme weather, it may take awhile. On those days when your spit freezes before it hits the ground, it's going to take you a long time just to get your core temperature to warm up at all, let alone all the muscles in your body. Remember that some warm up is better than no warm up at all. Do the best you can with your warm up. When you begin your exercise routine, start off slow, and then build your way up.

My example for this would be mountaineering. Some days mountaineers wake up at one or two o'clock in the morning to begin their ascent. It can be 20 degrees below zero, or even colder in some locations. The last thing these people want to do is jog in place or do some English Burpees to get ready to climb when they are at 20,000 feet elevation where breathing alone is a challenge. Mountaineers don't warm up because they just can't. It's too freaking cold! They start moving slowly and gradually pick up their pace. Eventually, they do get warmer if they are layered properly and do not stop moving.

Most importantly, listen to your body. If you feel a little kink in your knee or you notice that your back isn't quite right while warming up, you need to keep that in mind as you begin to get into your exercise routine. If the pain gets worse, you may want to call it quits for the day rather than injuring yourself. I always say, "It's better to under train and always train than to over train once". If you over train and injure yourself, you're done. Slightly under training allows you to continue your exercise routine pretty much year round with maybe one or two recovery weeks thrown in (competitive athletes are a different story, they need many recovery weeks in a year based on sport and program design).

Keep those layers handy, make sure you are warm before you begin to push yourself, and listen to your body when it speaks to you. Exercise is an addiction for some people and if it is taken away due to an injury, it can be both physically and mentally devastating. If this does happen, feel free to contact me; I know how to cope with this issue well.

I wish you the best of luck with your training. Be smart, train hard, and push your limits but don't exceed them - that's when injury occurs.

Take it up Two More Inches

I'm from a small town in Lake Tahoe called Zephyr Cove, which is on the Nevada side (it's pronounced Nevada not Nevawda) of Lake Tahoe. I attended George Whittell High School (250 students), and our cross-town rivals were the South Lake Tahoe High School Vikings (1,000 students). Even though they had four times as many students as we did, we still competed hard and often against them. In my prime, my glory days in high school, I was one of three stand-out athletes on our track team (I threw the discus). Our cross-town rivals also had their big three (one was a discus thrower, and I'm proud to say I never lost to him). At every meet, we would either compete against one another or watch the others compete. South Tahoe had a high jumper who was notorious for saying, "Take it up two more inches."

I recently had a client tell me that she felt like she would like to "raise the bar" on her training, and this got me thinking about that high jumper. He always wanted a challenge, even though there was a chance that he could fail. He wasn't afraid of failure; he knew that if he didn't put everything he had on the line, he would never succeed. I know a few people who are afraid of failure, and I'm here to encourage you not to be.

Michael Jordan once said, "I missed 100 percent of the shots I never took." You have to take a chance to provide yourself with the opportunity to succeed. That is my message for today. Don't be afraid of failure, as it can only make you stronger. Take a chance, raise the bar, and go for it. This can be applied to anything in life - a business opportunity, a new marketing strategy, or a new exercise program. Doing the same old exercises will produce the same old results. If those results are not what you are looking for, then it is time for a change. If you are due for a change, make it a big one!

Now, don't take my words out of context. If you have been walking two miles a day for six months, I don't want you to start running wind sprints. Pick a new challenge the next level up, and raise the bar to what is next in line for you. If you have been working out on the machine circuit for three months, then it might be time to learn some free weight exercises. If you have been taking step aerobics classes for a year and you are frustrated because your body hasn't changed much, look for a high intensity training group to join. I've said it before and I'll say it again, "Don't be afraid to be strong!" Challenge yourself by taking your stagnant routine to the next level, raise the bar!

* A special thank you goes out to a great friend and a wonderful client who inspired this chapter. Thank you Julie!

The Human Head Weighs Eight Pounds

I'm a huge fan of the movie "Jerry Maguire" and, of course, the title of this newsletter is a quote from that cute little kid with the glasses in the movie. As a personal trainer, I begin to notice certain trends over the years with my clients. One major trend I have noticed is the lack of neck strength in my female clients. I ask my clients to perform exercises like muscularly inverted (upside down) hangs with their feet up on a bench and their hands on a bar or a pair of gymnastic rings with their elbows flexed and shoulders slightly adducted to keep the joints strong (they are parallel with the floor). As they hold this position (great for core strength), they begin to either drop their heads back (dangling toward the floor) or they flex their necks trying to look at their belly buttons. It becomes difficult, even for men, to hold their heads perfectly straight or, in this case, parallel to the floor. As with any trend I discover, I have done some research on it and have found some information that I find rather interesting.

I stumbled across a study in which the study's administers bound participants' hands and then had them fall backward onto a wrestling mat (WWE wrestling mat, not the hard wrestling sport mats used in the Olympics). The administers observed the participants' heads as they hit the mat to see if they obtained the required amount of neck strength to keep their heads from hitting the mat. Nine out of ten men were successful in not hitting their head, but all ten women failed. The testing group was rather small; however, the male subjects all shared one meaningful similarity. All ten men had been or were still active in a sport which included the neck muscles being used in a contact prevention manner. These sports included rugby, football, soccer, and wrestling.

In contrast, most of the women participated in non head-contact sports, such as gymnastics, volleyball and basketball. This caused me to think about the muscles developed during teenage years, and how that set baseline strength for the neck in the years to come. The aforementioned sports are all offered to boys at a very young age. Years of participation in any of these sports, football in particular, would help to develop these neck muscles more than would other non head-contact sports. I remember when I played football in high school, we did neck strengthening exercises every day in the weight room and during our warm up prior to hitting drills.

Women, on the other hand, are not typically offered the opportunity to participate in these sports with exception to soccer as a seasonal or year round sport. Some schools did or still do offer females the opportunity to participate in wrestling, but the number of female participants is very small, meaning that females mostly wrestle against males. I would venture to guess that these females (soccer and wresting athletes) would have been more successful in this test.

The message I took from this research is this: neck muscles are like any other muscles in the body. They need to be trained in order to stay strong. Simply supporting the head in standing or seated positions is not enough work for the neck muscles over the average person's life span. There are some problems that can arise as a result of poor neck strength, including "forward head". "Forward head" normally occurs as a result of and is usually accompanied by poor posture. Many elderly individuals develop this posture (round upper back and head pushed forward) from years of poor posture, weak neck muscles, or over development of the anterior muscles of the neck, which results in the unnatural pulling of the head forward.

For the sake of your posture and your head and neck health, you may want to include some simple exercises to work on your neck strength. One basic exercise is performed by getting down on all fours (hands and knees) and slowly raising the head up toward the ceiling and holding for three seconds followed by slowly returning the neck to the neutral position for a set of ten repetitions. Remember this: the old saying "No pain no gain" does apply to the neck and back. If you have any pain, stop right away or you will not gain anything other than a trip to the doctor. As with any activity, be sure you have permission from your doctor to participate. Start out with one set of 10 every other day or so and build up slowly.

Injuring your neck can be devastating. Take precaution now and get the muscles of your neck strong, especially if you are a female, and work hard on correcting your posture. Proper posture breathes confidence and, in my opinion, looks more attractive. If not for my father constantly reminding me to "stand up straight, shoulders back" when I was growing up, I would likely have awful posture today. Just like anything, this will take time. Be patient, work smart, and improve yourself starting today.

I Can't Talk About It

Prior to your first session with your personal trainer, you decide to go to a local supplement shop to stock up on daily vitamins and protein bars. While you are in the store deciding which type of whey protein to buy, you are approached by the company "specialist" who asks if he can assist you. In most cases, this individual's education and experience with nutrition is based on reading "Flex" magazine and watching the movie *Pumping Iron*. There are many other professionals from whom you could instead receive this information, and one of them should be your personal trainer. Please pay special attention to that word "should" that I used in that last sentence.

As a personal trainer, I have spent the last 11 years of my life educating myself on nutrition and exercises. I have a master's degree in personal training. However, legally I am not permitted to speak to my clients about nutrition because I am not a certified dietitian or nutritionist. This rule stands for every personal trainer in the business, although it does not stop some trainers from doing so. The uneducated muscle-head at the vitamin store can give you nutritional advice after three hours of on-the-job training, but after earning a degree in kinesiology (study of the human body), I'm not even allowed to discuss it.

Other than a certified dietitian or nutritionist, who would be better educated to help you with your nutrition than your trainer? Quality personal trainers are extremely passionate about their jobs. They know how to exercise inside and out, and, better yet, they know all about nutrition and how vital your diet can be toward getting you into the physical condition you desire. I'm not talking about your low-end personal trainers who got their certifications in one day on the internet. I am talking about a personal trainer who has made a career out of training clients. I am talking about trainers who are certified through credible organizations (NSCA, ACSM, NASM, ACE or NFPT), who spend their own money going to clinics or seminars to learn more about their trade, and who wake up at four in the morning to prepare their workout programs for the day's clientele. This kind of trainer knows his or her craft, and should legally be allowed to speak to their clients about nutrition.

One major problem with the personal training business is that we are lacking a governing organization holding all trainers to a specified standard. If we had that organization and those standards by which to work, I believe that certified personal trainers would be allowed to give nutritional advice. Until that day comes, if you are currently receiving nutritional advice from your trainer, remember that legally they should not be providing you this information. If they are and you are accepting it, understand that they are breaking a law and if they are a true professional they will not discuss what they are not legally permitted to discuss. You need to find a trainer you can trust, who honors the code, and who is dedicated to the profession. When you find that person, you will have all the motivation, education and experience you need to achieve any fitness goal.

Do You Know What is SAID

The original *Rocky* film from 1976 (starring Sylvester Stallone, Burgees Meredith, Talia Shire, Carl Weathers and Burt Young - yes, I know all of the characters by both their real and character names from all six Rocky movies) is a story about a young man from the streets who aspires to become more than just a brawler. In the movie, the sport of boxing is called "the sweet science" because there is great strategy combined with general toughness in the sport. In one scene, Rocky increases his toughness by punching meat hanging on a hook. In fact, he punches the meat so hard that you can even hear the ribs breaking each time he hits it (true story - no sound effects - Stallone really did that!).

The part I want to focus on is the "punching the meat" scene. In the personal training field, we work by a couple of general training principles, and one is called the SAID principle. SAID stands for Specific Adaptations to Imposed Demands. In the rib cracking scene, Rocky is shown with his hands taped while smacking the meat around. If the average person (non-boxer) tried to perform this feat, he or she would cause serious damage to their hand and/or wrist. Due to the extreme volume of punches thrown during the average day of a boxer's training cycle, the bones in the hands and wrists begin to grow thicker. This thickness is a Specific Adaptation of the bone due to the Demand the boxer has Imposed on the bone by throwing so many punches per workout.

Gradually, over time, the wrists and hands become stronger both in bone density and muscularity, making this individual more adapted to the sport of boxing. The SAID principle can be applied to every muscle, bone, and movements. Any muscle placed under a load (demand) will grow in size (adapt) to overcome it. Women who consistently carry their child in the same hand and place them on the same hip develop a more muscular arm (isometrically speaking) and a "staggered hip." This is noticeable to the naked eye when observing a mother during her everyday routine. The stronger hip will consistently take precedence over the other and the stronger arm will be used more often to pick up or hold things compared to the other.

Take some time during your workout routine to think about the SAID principle and what you are doing to your body. SAID is not necessarily a bad thing; think of the boxer who needs that bone density and strength in the wrist to be able to punch that meat over and over again. For the demands placed on the boxer, this principle has worked greatly in his favor. Hand calluses from weightlifting and increased curvature of the spines of rowing athletes (not a good example, but an example nonetheless) are other examples of the SAID principle.

Embrace the SAID principle, as it can point out weaknesses in some areas of your body and develop strengths in others. Train hard, but remember to always train smart!

Backing up the Tripod

You can always spot a person with a bad back. They have a distinct walk with their hips slightly out, a very slight limp, and near perfect posture. I am one of those people, and I have all of these symptoms due to my lack of a strength and conditioning coach during my hammer throwing career. I practiced many poor lifting techniques over a ten year throwing career which eventually left my back permanently damaged. I like to think that my injury has made me a better personal trainer because I am always concerned about my clients' lifting techniques and the positioning of their hips. It has been four years since my back injury, and over that time I have developed a simple technique that has helped my back dramatically. It's called the "tripod" position.

This is a very simple technique I use any time I am moving weights around on the floor, working in my yard, or playing with my dog. I have both knees and one hand on the ground. Both knees are a given. No one with a bad back would choose to take one knee and twist while bending over; they will almost always go to both knees to work on the ground. The addition of the hand is the key part. The pressure of holding the weight of the torso is dramatically decreased in the lower back when a hand is placed on the ground. Think of kneeling down on the ground on all fours. When you place your body down on all fours and use one hand to perform a task, the weight of the torso is distributed, reducing the pressure on the lumbar and placing more of the load on the muscularity of the arms and legs. Yes, it may look a little odd to be the person crawling around on all fours pulling weeds in the yard, but you will be saving your back.

Back pain, if you have ever had it, is something you know you do not want to live with for the rest of your life. There are some techniques that can dramatically improve lower back pain, however odd they may look, as well as increase your quality of life. My advice to my fellow back pained individuals is to invest in a nice pair of knee pads. The tripod position, over a long period of time, can bring on some knee pain, and the last thing you want is to exchange the pain in your back for pain in your knees. If you are active in working around your house or keeping up the yard, knee pads can go a long way. A $30 investment to live a life with less back pain is a great exchange from my perspective.

When I was a kid, I was big into hero movies. I loved watching action movies like *Rocky*, *Rambo* and *The Terminator*. I often thought to myself, "What hero would I be if I could become one?" Today, I would be known as the "Tripod," healing backs all across the nation. After experiencing serious back pain, I wish it upon no one and only hope that my information can help reduce the pain that I have known oh-so-well. Take care of your back; you only get one. I often say to my clients, "Your back is like an electrical cord, it can bend and twist for years and then one day it will just snap." Please hear this advice, and think about the positioning of your back when you are putting on your shoes. Think about squatting down to pick up your kids and keep pushing yourself to improve your posture, as there is no such thing as "perfect". Protect your back in all that you do. If you ever need me, just yell out "tripod" and I'll be there!

Motivation: Training When You Don't Want To

Life gets in the way. It happens to all of us. We have plans to get up early and go to the gym every morning this week and start getting our bodies into better shape. Something comes up with work or with the family on Tuesday night, and when Wednesday morning comes around, we do not feel like getting up and pushing ourselves. Workloads increase, daily life becomes stressful, or we just commit to too many things. Whatever the reason, we all have the same feeling at times: "I don't want to train today." As a certified personal trainer, it is my duty to help you and all of my clients find that day-to-day motivation to stay the course. I have a few tips that may help you out.

Force yourself. I heard of a client who was so poorly motivated to go to the gym every evening after work that she would pack her gym bag and drive to the gym on her way to work in the morning. She would check in, drop off her bag with her house key in it, and proceed to work, thus forcing her to come back to get her house key if she wanted to go home. She knew that once she was literally "inside" the gym that she would then stay and do her workout. All she needed was an extra push to get her foot inside the door. Once inside, she knew she would decide to work out and feel good about it. After some time, she no longer needed to drop off her keys in the morning as she began to look forward to her evening workouts and made the gym a regular stop on her way home each night.

Think about your image. Recently, one of my clients brought me a picture of what she wanted her arms and chest to look like. This was my inspiration for the "Finding My Perfect Body" newsletter which started this whole thing. She saw a picture of this woman in a fitness magazine and was inspired by it. "I want my arms to look like this," she said to me as we began to create her program design. Similarly, I used to tape pictures of Arnold Schwarzenegger in my workout journal for inspiration. I have a client who keeps a picture of Madonna's ripped arms on the back of her sun visor in her car.

I worked with a young man who wanted his shoulders to look like Dwight Howard's. Whatever the look is that inspires you, keep it present in your life and continue to work toward it. You will never be able to look exactly like these other people as we are all built differently; however, in some cases, you could end up looking even better than the photos or images you select!

Power of the Mind. Since I was 13 years old, I have always been able to eat an entire large pizza by myself with no problem at all. Until recently, I had never associated any negative feelings with eating pizza at any stage of my life. I read a book called *The Female Body Breakthrough*, by Rachel Cosgrove. In her book, she discusses the mental association of negative feelings with a physical act. I ended up applying this strategy to my poor eating habits. I paid particular attention to the way I felt after eating pizza one day and discovered how heavy and crappy I felt. I locked this feeling into my mind. Since that day, I have had pizza once over the last three months.

I took two bites of a slice about a month into my change and felt sick. My mental connection with pizza has completely changed my eating habits, and I no longer desire it at all. This same mental connection can be made with the feelings of euphoria that come after a good workout. After your next great workout, focus your mind on how good you feel at that very moment. Lock that feeling in your mind, and learn to desire it. If you can do this for 21 days in a row, you can break or create any habit. No more negative associations like "I *have* to go workout". Instead, create a mindset like, "I *get* to go workout". The mind is a powerful thing if you are willing to utilize it beneficially and put forth a solid effort.

These techniques are just a few ways we can use to find the desire to train every day. Whatever your goal may be, twice a week, five times a week, or 30 minutes every day, you must take the necessary steps both physically and mentally to set yourself up for success. We are all too busy, we all have too much to do, and none of us has time in our regular routine unless we make it a priority. If it is important to you, you will find the time to do it! You can do it, and when times get tough, it's never too late to start your consecutive training streak again.

I'm Prepared to Die on a Treadmill

Over this last weekend, I was on my mentor's website when I saw a video he posted called, "Are you prepared to die on a treadmill?" I was just as curious as you were when you saw my heading for this newsletter, so I clicked on the link and it brought me to a video of Will Smith prior to the release of his movie "I Am Legend" (which is my favorite Will Smith movie - he does at least 15 behind the neck pull ups - it's totally awesome!). Will talks about how he does not want to be an icon as much as he wants to be an idea. He wants people to believe in themselves and constantly strive for the next step, the next chapter in their lives, or the next challenge.

At the end of the interview, he says, "I'm prepared to die on a treadmill," and explains that there is no way anyone is going to outwork him. No matter how strong or how endured they are, they are not going to work harder than he is and that he is, in fact, prepared to die on that treadmill to outwork the next person. I found extreme motivation in this statement, and wanted to share it all with you, as it pertains both to our fitness training and to our business commitments. Why would we want to be anything less than the best?

From day one, I have wanted to become the most educated, trusted and experienced personal trainer that the United States has to offer and that is something toward which I have dedicated over a decade of work. Would you, as the client, want to work with someone who wouldn't make that statement? Would you settle for mediocrity? I hope your answer is no, because I wouldn't.

I would want to work with the best, or with a committed person who wants to be the best. I want to work with the person who is prepared to go the distance, to push the limit, to sacrifice their time, and to die on that treadmill. This message goes for any aspect of life as well as for any business out there. It is not survival of the fittest anymore; it's survival of the most committed.

This idea can be applied to our health and fitness training. Challenge yourself during your next workout. Push yourself to the next level, because it will pay off for you as you get closer to achieving your goal. Don't settle for mediocrity. Challenge yourself to reach the next stage of your fitness training.

In the famous words of Apollo Creed (*Rocky I, II, III, IV*), "There is no tomorrow!" Don't put off your training until the next day. Do it now! Step up! Take the challenge, because if you don't, you will never know what you could have become. It's okay to fail; I've done it a million times. But it's not okay to give up. That is the beauty of our fitness training. It is never too late to start again.

My message is this: don't wait until tomorrow. Take that all-important step today and build off of it. If you take a step backwards, it's okay. The next day, you can move forward again. I ask you this: Are you prepared to die on that treadmill? Are you prepared to push yourself to the next stage of your fitness? We all have this idea of how hard we can push ourselves. If you push yourself just slightly over that "limit" each day, you can create the body you have always wanted. It may not happen today or tomorrow or next week or even next year, but if you truly believe and are truly dedicated to your cause, it will happen for you. It's like cutting down an oak tree; you have to take it one consistent swing at a time, and eventually you will achieve your goal.

Ice or Heat - Which One Does What and Why

We live in a fitness marketing society in which companies direct their marketing strategies at average Americans, assuming they have not doing their homework and trust the ad they have just seen or read about. The best example I can give you is Icy Hot. Icy Hot has NBA star Shaquille O'Neal as their spokesperson, and in their commercial, he is hard at work practicing his slam dunk. When he is done, he reaches for his back. The pain is too much for him to handle, so he puts on the Icy Hot patch that makes it all feel better. This is marketing at its best. However, I'm sorry to say that it is the worst possible thing you can do to your body at that point in time. I hear about my clients who feel muscles pull while they're out running, throw their backs out lifting up boxes over the weekend, or feel pains in their shoulders playing catch with their kids. No matter the injury or how it is obtained, the last thing you want to do is apply heat to it. By "heat", I mean an actual heating pad or any ointment that you can rub on your body, like Tigerbalm, Icy Hot, Bengay or Biofreeze. Don't fall into their marketing traps - here is the reason why.

The best way I can explain it is by using the freeway as an example. When you are driving on the freeway and there is no traffic, you can't really see anything around you because you are moving by so quickly. A lot of damage could be done to an object you hit because you are moving so fast. When you apply heat to an injured muscle, the heat brings blood flow to that area quickly. The damaged muscle now has a mass amount of blood moving very fast directly to and around the injured area. The blood is much like the car on the freeway in that it is going to cause more damage to the muscle because it is moving so quickly. Imagine this mass amount of blood pushing through a torn muscle. It will simply continue to tear the muscle because there is an overabundance of blood rushing to that area. Heat was originally created for tight muscles, not for injured muscles. If you wake up every morning with a tight back or hip flexor, applying heat is the way to go. You want blood to flow to that area, as it loosens up the tight muscle. This does not create any damage because there is no preexisting injury there.

Ice, on the other hand, causes a major traffic jam. There are cars everywhere, and no one is moving quickly at all. As the blood flow to the area slows down, the white blood cells have enough time to start fixing the injured area because they are not hurried out by a massive blood flow behind them. The ice slows the blood flow and the white blood cells begin to heal this injured area. Twenty to thirty minutes of ice applied to an injured area will help the injured muscle to repair itself. There is no such thing as icing too much, as long as you don't exceed thirty minutes and allow thirty minutes between application periods. As you ice, the muscle will get cold and stiffen up a bit. Taking the extra thirty minutes between icing will allow the muscle to warm up a little before starting the healing process over again. This is why athletes sit in ice buckets after a hard practice or game. The muscles are beat up and sore. The ice encourages the healing process however painful it may be for the first few minutes.

I tell people, "Make it through the first three minutes and you will be fine. You won't even feel it anymore." It's true. Once you get through the first three minutes, you are golden. One other hard part about icing is how unpleasant it is when you are already cold. It is March, and it's very cold outside. None of us wants to willingly place ice around our bodies when it's 65 degrees or less in the house. I make it a habit, no matter what, to ice my back every night as I go to bed. I have a large ice pack that is molded into a belt which I wrap around my back before I hop in to bed. It stays cold for about thirty minutes and, at some point during the night, I wake up and take it off quickly. I wake up feeling good every morning.

My message is this: if you have an injury, don't put heat on it, ever! If you have a tight muscle, alternate between ice and heat every hour. This will create healing opportunities, and will loosen up the muscle. When in doubt, use ice! I know it may not be the most comfortable thing, but it works. I guarantee it! Stop wasting your money on those ointments. Invest in some ice packs and heal your body up right.

CPT Business: Separating yourself as an Elite Personal Trainer
(Published in On Fitness Magazine July/August 2011 – Volume 11 Issue 7)

There are many successful, hard working and dedicated certified personal trainers in the fitness industry. The one trait that every one of them shares is passion. A passionate professional wakes up each morning and looks forward to getting to work that day. The energy he or she brings to clients and co-workers is infectious, and continues to grow with each passing year.

The elite level certified personal trainers are deeply passionate about their work, and often take steps toward improving themselves. They are eager to learn, and are very successful with their clients, with their business, and with life in general. The field within the fitness industry in which these trainers specialize does not matter. All that matters is that they are constantly trying to improve themselves, the quality of their product and the positive effects they have on their clients.

How do you distinguish yourself as one of these elite level certified personal trainers in the fitness industry today? By following these three steps. They will assist you in getting started down the right path.

Certify and affiliate with a reputable organization
There are many certifying organizations in the fitness industry; however, only a handful of them are nationally recognized. The elite certifying organizations want to place their initials after the names of dedicated, passionate and well-educated fitness professionals.

That is why many of these organizations require a certain level of completed education prior to allowing a participant to register for a certification exam, purchase their study materials, or simply to become a member of the organization.

The elite certifying organizations (listed below) hold their fitness professionals to a certain standard once their certifications have been obtained. Continued education units (CEUs) are required by the certifying organization to ensure that their representatives are making every effort to further educate themselves.

Unprofessional personal trainers view meeting these required number of CEUs as a bother. Elite level certified personal trainers see this requirement as an opportunity to build their education, to learn new training techniques, to hear about new research in a fitness field that is constantly changing, and to advance themselves professionally.

Some elite certifying organizations include:
- The National Strength and Conditioning Association (NSCA)
- American College of Sports Medicine (ACSM)
- American Council on Exercise (ACE)
- National Academy of Sports Medicine (NASM)
- National Federation of Professional Trainers (NFPT)
- USA Weightlifting (USAW)

Become the specialist.
The client wants to know that he or she is in good hands. Often, when someone goes to the hospital, she sees a specialist for almost any symptom she experiences. Seeing a certified personal trainer should not be any different. There are many fields within the fitness industry in which a certified personal trainer can specialize. Boot camps, strength training, fat loss, body building, corrective exercise, Olympic lifting, group training, core training, power lifting, endurance training, program design and functional movement screening, just to name a few, are areas of specialization that can be selected.

Once a specific field has been selected, the trainer should make every effort to market him or herself as much as possible as the specialist in that field. Emails, text messages, newsletters, fliers, business cards, and websites are a few marketing tools in which the trainer's name and specialty should be paired together.

The trainer's goal is to be known as "the person to go to" for the specific area of focus. Many trainers are afraid to specialize, and feel that it pigeonholes them into working within only a certain demographic of clientele. There are many examples of successful certified personal trainers in the fitness industry today who have focused their skills in one particular area. These successful individuals have committed themselves to being the best at one specific area rather than being mediocre in multiple fields. This doesn't mean they are not well-rounded; however, they are exceptional in their respective areas of focus. The fitness industry is massively evolving right now, and becoming a "specialist" is part of that evolution.

Some specialists in the fitness industry include:
- Alwyn Cosgrove: Fat loss
- Gary Cook: Functional movement
- Mike Boyle: Strength coach
- Todd Durkin: Mindset and motivation
- Rachel Cosgrove: Female body image
- Lee Burton: Corrective exercise
- Stuart McGill: Lower back injuries

Do more than train your clients; also consult with them.
There is a special relationship that develops between a client and a trainer who work really well together. It is a relationship built on the trust, faith and commitment that each has in the other. The relationship will thrive and goals will be achieved as long as both participants pull their weight. One way trainers can ensure they are doing their part is to consult with the client.

Scheduling monthly or quarterly meetings where the trainer can meet with the client to discuss progress, program design, and eating and hydrating habits as well as re-evaluate the client's goals helps the trainer to better assist the client's continual improvement. Clients love to be spotlighted and have a discussion solely based around them and their training routine, and trainers who show this extra bit of effort often get referred to more prospective clientele. Nothing sounds better to a trainer than hearing his or her clients are so pleased with their experiences that they are now referring other business.

Elite certified personal trainers take the time to communicate with their clients and make sure they are happy with the quality of their product, which in turn leads to more referrals. They send out emails, text messages or surveys asking their clients how they can improve. The feedback received is vital to the future of the trainer's business, and it shows the client that their opinion has value.

Every certified personal trainer should want to take his or her business and the quality of the product to the next level. Certifying and affiliating with a reputable organization, becoming a specialist in a specific fitness field, and consulting with clients will assist the trainer in distinguishing him or herself as one of the elite individuals in the business.

Poor Man's Massage

Many of my clients have been asking me why we foam roll before or after a workout. There are many reasons why we do this, and the first one I want to discuss is that it feels good. I have said in the past that just because it feels good doesn't mean that it's good for your body. I have a few ladies who love to round their backs over and reach toward the floor because it "feels good" on their lower backs. Doing this "stretch" damages the lumbar and can lead to serious injury. I like to joke and say, "I'm sure LSD feels good, but it's not good for your body," meaning that some things that we do to our body may feel pleasurable but can actually cause a lot of damage.

In the case of the foam roller, it is not damaging as long as you are using it correctly. It does feel rather good, especially for us lower back issue folks, to roll out and massage those tight muscles. The famous "IT" band is the one that doesn't feel all that great, but the result of dealing with that pain over times can reduce severe hip, knee, and shin pain. Foam rolling is a major contributor to your blood flow because it works much like a suction device. It has been proven that if you stand with your knees locked for an extended period of time without moving, you will pass out. The reason for this is the lack of blood flow back up to your brain. When you move your legs (even swaying back and forth), the muscles act as a suction device by contracting in a "rolling" fashion to pressure the blood in the legs back up to the heart.

The foam roller performs a similar function. As you roll a muscle from top to bottom, you are creating pressure which pushes blood out. That blood being pushed out causes an increase in blood return to that same area. You are creating a freshly oxygenated blood flow to the area you are rolling.

Studies have tested resting heart rate compared to the heart rate when performing the simple roll on the lower back. Naturally, they found that a participant's heart rate was slightly higher while foam rolling because the person was moving. Interestingly, there was a higher increase in heart rate when performing the foam roll on the lower back because more blood was being pressured back to the heart. In turn, the heart had to pump more blood to keep that blood flow moving.

Foam rolling, on most body parts, feels good, and it increases blood flow and flexibility. On the other hand, there is NO scientific evidence that suggests that static stretching (stretch and hold for thirty seconds) increases flexibility. However, evidence does suggest that dynamic stretching increases flexibility. Dynamic stretching includes moving muscles through an increasing range of motion while continuing motion. One example is the walking lunge. Each lunge causes stretching of the back leg's hip flexor and the front leg's gluteus. Repeating full range of motion lunged increases flexibility to those two muscles. Foam rolling is a form of dynamic stretching, as you are moving the muscle in a range of motion that the muscle does not normally perform.

There is only one way to stretch a muscle, and that is by elongating it. Let's take the quadriceps as an example. When you grab your foot and pull it up toward your butt, you are elongating your quadriceps to stretch them. The foam roller elongates the muscle without having to move it. The roller pushes the muscle inward creating a very slight elongation of the muscle. The muscle is not used to this because we rarely perform something like this day to day, but this slight elongation of the muscle being pushed in can drastically increase the muscle's flexibility. This increased flexibility leads to reduced pain in the joints (most famous for this is the "IT" band).

The foam roller is a great tool, but, like all tools, can be detrimental if overused. A few minutes each day will work wonders; just don't overdo it! Here is a basic foam rolling routine I have my clients perform called "The 100." I also like to call it the "Poor Man's Massage!"

10 Rolls to Each Body Part: 40 each leg = 80 Total
Gluteus (Butt)
Hamstring
Hip Flexor
IT Band

10 Rolls to the Back: 10 each section of back = 20 Total
Upper Back
Lower Back

Row Your Way Strong

I am currently in Valencia (Southern California) attending a seminar with my mentors, Rachel and Alwyn Cosgrove. Over the last few months, my clients' requests for "personalized program designs" have dramatically increased. I'm thrilled about this because I love writing programs! I have studied program design since 1999 and have loved it from the beginning. The thing I like most about program design is that a self-motivated person can get to the gym and push herself with a professionally developed workout program designed for her fitness needs without a trainer present.

When you think about it, there are 168 hours in a week, and I get to see most of my clients for two of them. If I could have them performing my workouts the other days of the week, their success rates in accomplishing their fitness goals would go way up. What I want most is for my clients to be successful and achieve something. This three day seminar that I am attending is designed to teach me more about program design. So all you program design followers out there, be ready! I'm coming home with new material!

The majority of the programs that I create involve using rowing machine for a warm-up. A couple of my clients have asked me why I like the rowing machine so much, and my answer is this: the rowing machine warms up every muscle and every joint in the human body in a very efficient manner. It's a non-impact exercise that almost everyone can participate in, even bad back folks like me. If you examine the exercise called the "dead-lift high pull," you will notice that it is the exact same movement as the rowing machine only performed vertically. The pressure on the spine and hips performing the high pull may be too much for some to handle; therefore, placing them on the rowing machine is just as efficient and allows for little to no tension on the spine and hips if performed correctly.

There are two ways to row, American style and European style. The American style is performed by rounding the back over and reaching as far forward as possible. This style is very hard on the lower back, but it produces good results as far as efficiency (meters per pull) is concerned. The European style of training keeps the back arched at all times and provides a constant contact to the chain of pull. This allows for immediate power production but does not produce as many meters per pull.

So which one is better? When looking over the results from the last four years of world competitions, the Americans have lost all but one race (women's eight person - Olympic Gold 2008). In theory, the American style provides a longer pull, but the pull is not as powerful as the European style pull. It is a more powerful and a more bio-mechanically sound position from which to pull. That is why I teach my clients to row like the Europeans.

Performing a small amount of rowing every day will eventually make your body stronger. Start by rowing 500 meters. This should take you anywhere between one and a half and four minutes, depending on your cardiovascular shape. Remember, it's not about how many pulls you can perform; it's about how powerful each pull can be. I remind my clients that the rowing machine should sound like the ocean when being used. You should hear a wave and then nothing, another wave and then nothing. If you are hearing wave after wave after wave with no break, you are rowing too fast. Keep your good posture, and don't be afraid to ask a trainer to help you with your technique. This is an exercise you must learn and practice in order to perform it more efficiently. After a week or so of rowing 500 meters each day, take it up to 800 meters. Over time, as your technique and condition improve, you can increase your meters up to 2,000. Anything more than this, on a daily basis, may be overdoing it. Get out there and row your body strong. Remember, keep that chest up and back arched!

50% Fitness Success Rate if You...

I recently asked one of my clients to transfer from her private one-on-one training sessions to a semi-private group training class. I informed her that she was physically ready for the next step in her training and that she would, in fact, receive a better workout when training with others. She asked me why training with other people would produce better results than training privately, and this is what I told her. In the late 1890s, a man named Norman Tripplett discovered something he called "social facilitation" through a series of tests performed on cyclists. Social facilitation is the naturally occurring competitive drive that an individual produces when in the presence of others. Think about the last time you had a push-up competition with your wife, husband, child, sister, brother or friend. Did you perform more push-ups when others were watching you than you would have on your own? If your answer is yes, then you have experienced social facilitation.

The personal training business is historically built on social facilitation. My profession was developed in the 1950s, a time when lifting weights was considered weird. Against all odds, a weight lifting fanatic named Jack LaLanne took the personal training business national when he aired "The Jack LaLanne Show" on ABC in 1959. The success of this show kept Jack on TV for over 34 years, a success which transformed once gym rats who gave orientations for free monthly dues into "fitness professionals." Personal training as a profession developed from the days of Reg Park, Bill Pearl, Larry Scott, Arnold Schwarzenegger, Frank Zane and Lee Haney. These body builders were the kings of a very small society of body building fanatics that, over time, evolved into a worldwide craze.

The 1980s brought, in addition to Madonna, acid washed jeans and side ponytails, a fitness craze focused around action movie stars like Schwarzenegger, Stallone, Eastwood, Willis and Van Damm. The personal training business was at an all-time high, and private one-on-one training was considered the way to go if you wanted results. The 1990s rolled around and nothing much changed in the business, other than personal trainers having to become "certified" and continually educate themselves in order to keep their certifications. I am not sure when the semi-private group strength training trend began, but it happened for me in 2004. This when I learned about and witnessed first-hand the concept of social facilitation. I began training multiple clients at once, and watched as my clients dramatically changed their bodies in much less time. I started urging my one-on-one clients to try training with a partner or two. Suddenly, I had half of my schedule filled up with groups.

This was the reasoning behind my developing a personal training studio. Other trainers and club members grew tired of my clients dominating all the equipment in the main gym. Now, in my own facility, I have 80% of my schedule filled with groups. 15% of my clients are slowly improving with the hopes of some day moving into a group, and 5% want to stay private. I am a man of my word, as all certified personal trainers should be, and will keep my private clients solo until they are ready. However, my goal is for all of my clients to eventually be training in groups.

Not buying it just yet? Listen to this statistic. As of 2009, the success rate of the private one-on-one personal training clients achieving their fitness goals was a whopping 3%. By contrast, clients training in semi-private groups have a 51% chance of achieving their goals, and that number is climbing! The proof is in the pudding. If you have the opportunity, try out a semi-private group strength training class, take advantage of it as it can change your life. Do not get this confused with step aerobics or spin class; make sure your class is semi-private group strength training.

Your instructor should teach you how to over head squat, swing kettle bells, perform push-ups and do pull-ups. Don't be intimidated by movements like these, or by training in front of others. They will each make you fitter, healthier and more resistant to injury. If you are sick of the same old results, get out there and try training with others. If you do, I guarantee one thing: you will have a much better chance of achieving your goals!

A special thank you goes out to Jack LaLanne, who passed away earlier this year. He was the "godfather" to personal trainers everywhere and single handedly paved the way for the rest of us in the personal training business. Thank you, Mr. LaLanne, for all that you have done. Without you and your efforts, we would not be where we are today.

Ditch the Cardio

Have you seen the movie *Terminator II: Judgement Day*? Linda Hamilton plays Sarah Conners, the mother of John Conners, who is the future leader of the revolution against the machines. Linda, preparing to work opposite Arnold Schwarzenegger, trained hard in the weight room to get her body to look the part necessary to represent such a strong character. In a magazine article she talks about how much weight training she did to get her body into shape. The columnist was surprised to find that she didn't do any cardiovascular exercise at all. Here is how she did it.

When you get on the treadmill or go outside for a run, your body moves at the same pace for an average amount of time. For example, say you go on a five mile run during which you hold 10 minute miles. Your body knows it has to work at this 60% effort for 50 minutes to complete this exercise. Repeating this same cardiovascular exercise multiple times during the week trains your body to go into "starvation mode", meaning that the body will begin to store fat and burn it's most efficient energy, which is no longer fat. The body instead begins to burn muscle as energy. This over time achieves the result that everyone wants. You do lose weight and get smaller; however you are now what we call "skinny fat." You are thin and have no muscle. Additionally, you are weak and have a higher body fat percentage.

When training with weights, the heart rate is constantly jumping up during and just after a set and then lowering back down during rest periods. This interval training style spikes your metabolism, and can keep it going for two to three days after a workout. One hour on the treadmill leaves your metabolism running high for an hour or two. Linda Hamilton got her body lean and ripped by lifting weights, and not little three pound pink weights during step class. She worked out hard and lifted heavy weights. The heavier the weight, the better (as long as you use proper technique). Especially you ladies out there. Yes, I am saying to all of you women - you need to lift heavy weights to get leaner, stronger and in the best shape of your life!

"But I'll get too bulky!" No, you won't. Trust me; you don't have enough testosterone in your body to get "too" bulky. Yes, when you train a muscle that has not been trained before, that muscle will grow. Yes, when you start lifting weights, the muscle will get slightly bigger, but much stronger. Think about the girls you see on the covers of *Fitness Rx* or *On Fitness* magazines. These pictures are guaranteed not to be digitally enhanced. The way those women got in that kind of shape was by lifting heavy weights.

Don't be a "Cardio Queen"; lift some weights! I can't stress this enough. Men and women, you need to lift weights! It is so good for your body. Trust me, and if you don't, call me and I'll read to you all the "scientifically proven" material supporting my stance. If you are doing your thirty minutes on the Elliptical every day and your body looks the same as it has for the last three years, then it's time for a change! Thirty minutes of lifting weights six days a week can change your body dramatically with proper nutrition. Period. Notice I didn't say "and cardio" after that. You don't need cardio to get thin. I promise you that!

Get the body you have always dreamed of, and do it the right way. If you need help, email or call me. That is why I am here - to help you to achieve your goals. I can't impress this message enough: lift weights to get healthy, strong, thin, and sexy (and look better naked, that is the goal for all of us)! The best way to do that is by lifting weights. Spike that metabolism; it will burn fat for you all day long. Eat small meals consisting of one fruit, one vegetable, some healthy fat, and some clean protein every three hours or so. Eating more often will keep you from eating too much. Three square meals a day is not the right way to do it. Eat small, eat often, spike your metabolism, and lift your weights. If you are a cardiovascular athlete, then you use cardio to train for your event. If you want to look great, feel great and be in the best shape of your life, then you need to...come on, you can say it...yes! Lift weights!

The 9 Out of 10 Rule

Now I know I'm not supposed to talk about nutrition, but since I will very broad in my discussion I feel that I am within my professional setting to discuss it. The "nine out of ten" rule is something I picked up a few years ago from a nutritionist in Chico. Basically, it states that every nine out of ten meals you are going to eat should be a healthy meal. The tenth meal can include something fun, like ice cream, cake, or a high caloric drink. This rule allows you to experience the successes of eating well without totally removing those items you really enjoy.

To keep your metabolism high, you should eat every three hours. Hungry or not, every three hours. No matter what. This habit becomes more like a ritual because you need to have all the right pieces to perform it correctly. Generally speaking, a fruit, a vegetable, a clean protein, and a healthy fat are recommended as parts of every meal. Eating these healthy selections every three hours usually gives you five to six meals per day. If you are adhering to the nine out of ten rule, this means you get a "fun" meal every other day. If you think about it, that's not all that bad. I have had this idea in my head for the last couple of years and have never implemented it recently. Three weeks ago, I began following this eating pattern and have since lost eight pounds. This coming from a guy who only exercises three to four times a week for half an hour.

Proper nutrition is something that we all know we are *supposed* to have; the hard part is sticking to it. This meal pattern allows you to have those "fun" meals every other day, which is important because then you do not feel like you are depriving yourself. Notice that I did not call this a "diet". The term "diet" is used to describe a modified or limited style of eating. The true meaning of the word is "the food eaten daily". The term "diet" is used incorrectly by most; we don't start "new diets", we simply change our current diet.

Make healthy choices, and you will feel and sleep much better. Take it from me, Mr. Pizza, Ice Cream and Cake; unhealthy choices only make you feel sick and heavy after you eat them. Keep it down to once every other day or so. Before you know it, you won't even crave these things. I have said it before and I'll say it again: it takes 21 days to break a habit. You can do it! Change your diet today, and get moving in the right direction.

Fitness is Everywhere

I have always found the development of my profession to be interesting. For a long time, personal trainers were more commonly referred to as "meat heads" before they were required to have certifications. The term "meat head" implies that the person being referenced has no brain, but instead has extra muscle to take up the space where the brain should be (hence the term "meat head").

As personal trainers have evolved into certified and educated professionals, their working space has also developed. My wife and I recently took a trip to San Francisco to visit the famous Alcatraz Prison (one of my favorite movies of all time is Clint Eastwood's *Escape from Alcatraz* in which he and some inmates create fake heads and place them in their bunks at night to fool the guards). As we took the tour and wandered around, we came across the guards' quarters. On the sign it read, "Guards Quarters and Gymnasium". I was so excited to see that even the world's most famous prison had a gym for exercise. I took a look inside and found a crumbling old building slowly falling apart. But, I did see a pull-up bar still mounted to the side of a wall which gave me hope that even back in the 1950s and 60s, the guards on this island were exercising often.

Gyms back in the "old days" (50s - 70s) were small boxes that no one would admit they were a part of unless he was a body builder. Today, there are gyms everywhere, often giving me the feeling that we are being invaded by health and fitness. Exercise has always been a priority for people, dating back hundreds of years. In our day and age we have more gyms, shopping malls, strip malls and warehouses than any other country in the world. Yet, we still have the highest obesity levels for both adults and children. How can so many facilities be open to so many people without them taking advantage of it? Do they work out at home? Are they embarrassed to work out in front of other people? Is a gym membership too expensive for their monthly budget? The answers to all of these questions could be yes, although there is a specific answer for every one of them.

There is some fantastic home-based exercise equipment that can be purchased and mounted on the backs of doors or door frames in your house. The initial investment will be a bit large (150 to 500 dollars) but afterwards, your "home gym" will be ready to go at your convenience, each session free of charge.

There are also options for those of you who do not enjoy exercising in front of other people. For example, there is a gym called "Fitness Together", which has a one-to-one trainer to client ratio. The client and trainer work in a private facility for the client's entire session. Do I think this is the right way to train? Not at all; I think group training is the best option. However, many people appreciate one on one training, especially when first getting started, so it is good to know that this option exists for them.

Are gym memberships too expensive? Many facilities require an initial start-up fee and monthly dues after that. Starting at a gym can be very expensive, if you do not know what to look for. Most gyms, usually twice a year for one month, will waive the initial set-up fee and allow a potential member to join by paying only the low monthly dues required. Waiting for this opportunity can save you some money, but understand what that low monthly payment is getting you. Usually, not much. You are allowed access to the facility for $19.99 a month, but what else? Anything extra, well, that will cost you money.

There is no such thing as a deal that is "too good to be true". My father used to tell me that if it's too good to be true, it probably is. There is always a catch, so be sure to look for it. My message in this newsletter is to encourage members of our society to be active, and to do so by embracing every tool and opportunity there is. There is no better day than today to begin your new healthy lifestyle. There is no better day than today to start eating right and join a gym. There is no better day than today to get off the cardio machines and learn how to lift some weights to make a change to your body. Do not be afraid of these changes; embrace them, and welcome them into your mind and heart. It will change the way you look at life and the way you feel on a daily basis. Don't believe me? Ask people who exercise. Most likely, the best they will feel all day is right after exercising. Find a fitness activity that you enjoy, and be as consistent and dedicated to it as possible. I have met many people who say they have been exercising consistently for six months, and have not yet seen any improvements. If this is the case for you, I guarantee that you have room to make positive changes to your workout routine. The human body will change when it is physically challenged correctly.

Find a trainer whom you trust, and buy into them completely. Dive into a workout program, and stay consistent with it. Like I said, there is no better day than today to start your new healthy lifestyle! Go make a change for the better. Go make a change for your health. Go make a change for you and for those closest to you. I promise, it will all be worth it in the end. Make today a great day!

Is Stretching Bad For You?

Often in these newsletters, you read about something I call "old school" training. By "old school" training, I mean the "no pain no gain" type of mentality which maintains that if the exercise you are performing doesn't hurt, then it is not working. I had a client come in about six months ago asking for a program design. After our initial assessment, I created a program heavily emphasizing flexibility because I could that the participant's flexibility was very poor and needed the most attention.

I prescribed something called "dynamic stretching," or what we call the "SECS". This does not stand for South Eastern Conference (for you NCAA football fans); rather, it is an acronym for Scorpions, Eagles, Cats/Dogs and Seal dynamic stretches. These dynamic stretching exercises are performed on the floor, and consist of holding a stretch for up to three seconds, moving into another position and holding for three seconds, and finally moving back to the first position until the appropriate number of repetitions has been completed.

In our first session, I informed my client that her flexibility was a major priority and that I had created her program with the specific goal of improving it in mind. My client's immediate response was, "I don't want to stretch. I'm paying you to teach me to work out." Right away, I could see her "old school" mentality bursting out. After some encouragement, I talked my client into sitting down and stretching. The first thing she did was put one leg straight out on the floor in front of her and then folded the other one behind her hip (the old school hurdle stretch) and began bouncing toward the front straight leg toes with both hands. Immediately, I asked my client to stop. "Well, you told me to stretch!" Again, she exemplified the old school mentality at its best. This technique is called "ballistic stretching", and is performed by bouncing into stretch repeatedly, performing a pulsing motion rather than holding a stretch consistently. This style of stretching can create a very explosive muscle reaction. There are track and field coaches at very successful universities who encourage ballistic stretching because they want their sprinters and throwers to be very explosive in their events. However, this manner of stretching has high potential for muscle pulls and tears. With such great risk for injury, I do not advise anyone to practice it.

After explaining this to my client, she then reached, straight legged, out to her toes and held them. Again, I ask my client to stop. "You said don't bounce!" Oh boy, old school mentality; here we go again. This is called "static stretching", and has actually been proven not to increase flexibility. Holding a stretch for up to thirty seconds allows the muscle to relax and, in turn, to stretch out to a longer length. Once the stretcher returns the muscle to its normal position, it will return to its original length. Any muscle, once it has become warm, will increase in length. This is why Bikram Yoga has become so popular. I have many clients who participate in it regularly and swear that it has helped to improve their flexibility. Well, it has proven to be very relaxing and to increase joint strength, but not flexibility. A warm muscle is similar to a rubber band in that when it is stretches, it will loosen up. As the muscle cools back down to its original temperature, it tightens back up to its original length. At this point, it has not improved much, if at all.

"What do you want me to do, then?" my client barked at me. "If you will let me talk, I'll tell you," I replied. Needless to say, this did not go over well. After cooling down my client, I described and demonstrated some dynamic flexibility exercises (SECS) and then encouraged her to try them. Against her will, she finally gave in and began performing the eagle stretch. She then admitted, "This actually feels really good". I explained that the continuous motion of a muscle through a large range of motion repeatedly extends and shortens it throughout its full range. As the muscle begins to warm up, it also begins to increase in range of motion, similarly to what happens after completing other styles of stretching. The difference between traditional stretching methods and dynamic flexibility exercises is that the muscle fibers are asked to stretch and contract over and over again without a hold or a bouncing movement. Think again about the rubber band. If you stretch it and shorten it over and over again, eventually the fibers inside it will begin to "tear" (in a good way) and elongate. These "tears" are micro-tears, and are not harmful to the muscle if the stretching exercises are performed correctly. Over time, these tears allow the muscle to increase in length, in turn creating a more flexible muscle.

The message of the story is this: constant movement of a muscle through a full range of motion will increase flexibility. Once a muscle is warm, performing a movement under a load is even more productive. This means that if you perform a squat with your body weight and after warming up perform it again holding 30 pounds, the range of motion will slightly increase because gravity is pulling down the weight in your hands. This movement performed multiple times will therefore increase those muscles' flexibility. If you are interested in learning more about dynamic stretching, please contact your personal trainer, as it is not something I can describe easily in a newsletter.

So, is stretching bad for you? No. However, it is only beneficial if it is performed dynamically and correctly. My originally resistant client, the one who didn't want anything to do with stretching and kept barking at me every time I said something, is now one of my closest clients. Now, she performs her SECS daily prior to our workouts. She has seen a dramatic improvement in her flexibility. Still, to this day, she jokes about how much she hated me that first session.

This goes to show that there is still a little "old school" left in all of us. However, thanks to science, we have developed and discovered more efficient ways to strengthen and improve our bodies.

CPT Business: Education is the key to success
(Published in On Fitness Magazine July/August 2011 - Volume 11 Issue 7)

Every two or three years, we, as certified personal trainers, are required to earn a predetermined number of continued education units (CEU) to maintain our certification statuses. During every recertification period we sign up for classes, register for new certifications, or attend clinics, camps, conferences, seminars and symposiums. Opportunities like these are often offered, encouraging us to continue educating and advancing ourselves as fitness professionals.

So, why is it so important for us to earn those CEUs? There are multiple answers. The first is our need Constant Never Ending Improvement (CNEI). As Certified Personal Trainers (CPTs), we must look to continually educate ourselves to in turn improve the quality of product we provide. Secondly, networking with other CPTs and opportunities for career advancement come hand-in-hand with the CEU-earning process. Through symposiums, workshops, and classes related to the personal training profession, we should be encouraged to meet our peers, discuss fitness related topics, and potentially pursue new business endeavors. CEUs and the ways we go about perusing them can assist us in taking the next steps in our careers. Obtaining the required CEUs provides us with so many opportunities. However, we must go pursuing them with the appropriate mindset.

In our case (and many others), education is the key to success. To assist you in achieving that success and developing the proper mindset required to become a successful fitness professional, I would like to take a deeper look into these two categories I have described.

Constant Never Ending Improvement (CNEI)
The fitness industry constantly changes. What may have been the best way to train our clients five years ago may not be so today. Scientific studies and in-depth research have provided an abundance of evidence supporting or discrediting training techniques and program design associated with the personal training business. Learning, and later,

applying this relevant information can change the way we work with and the success we have with our current clientele.

Our clients put faith in us as fitness professionals to be up to date on the cutting edge information on physical fitness, and to be able to apply that information accordingly to program designs. Learning this information allows us to take our professional development to the next level. Continually adding to our educations will assist us in elevating both the quality of our products and the stature we have as certified personal trainers.

As professionals, it should be each of our goals to be known in the training facility as "the educated personal trainer" who knows the profession better than anyone else. Our clients value education, and feel more comfortable working with someone who continually makes an effort to educate him or herself. We have all heard the saying "knowledge is power". In this profession, this statement could not hold more truth.

Networking and Career Advancement
There are opportunities for us to network with other certified professionals in our field at every CEU event. Networking has many benefits. It allows us to develop professional relationships with our peers as well as to make potential career advancements. Networking can be as simple as discussing training techniques with others during a break between speakers at a clinic, or as prestigious as presenting at a CEU event.

Presenting allows you with the opportunity to spotlight yourself as a professional. It also enables you to share valuable information which can be used to improve other trainers' practices. Speaking at an event can be nerve-wracking, but it can assist you in bringing credibility to your name as a professional and could in turn lead to new business opportunities.

Many of us are looking to take that next step in our careers. You can initiate these first steps while networking with other fitness experts.

Establishing relationships with other professionals as a result of basic networking can lead to great opportunities, such as writing or co-writing a book, creating DVD instructional videos, or presenting at future CEU events.

Networking can go even further. You can establish future business partnerships, or get a jump-start on applying for a position with a desired company. The sky is the limit in our profession, and we should take every opportunity to meet and talk with our peers. You never know where a simple introduction might lead you. Exchanging business cards is a great way to stay in touch with other professionals and to leave a lasting impression on someone who could potentially advance your career.

Michael Jordan once said, "You miss 100 percent of the shots you never take". The message of this quotation well applies to our profession. Take every opportunity you can to meet other fitness professionals and to develop professional relationships, because you never know what opportunity you might be missing out on in future.

Passionate Mindset
In the personal training profession, it takes time to develop a committed and passionate mindset. Our first priority should be to assist our clients in achieving their fitness goals. You feel a great sense of accomplishment when you see the look on your client's face when she perform her first chin up, when he back squats his body weight, when she fits into her skinny jeans, or when any one of your clients meets his or her specific fitness goal.

As more of our clients begin achieving their goals, our passion for what we do should grow deeper. To continue to educate and improve our clients, we need to continue to educate and improve ourselves. Some trainers view the CEU requirement as a burden whereas the more passionate trainers view it as chance to bring new information back to their clients. These educational experiences teach us the keys to improving our own practices as we get to listen to experienced professionals discuss the steps they took in achieving their successes.

When it comes down to it, we should all be passionate professionals who constantly strive to improve our product and ourselves. We should be passionate professionals reaching out to our peers within our profession. We should be passionate professionals seizing any chance to advance our profession and our careers. Simply put, we should be passionate professionals trying to make a difference.

Fitness Networking

As I write this email, I am sitting in the McCarran International Airport in Las Vegas, waiting for my flight back home to Sacramento. My wife and I have spent the last three days in Las Vegas participating in the National Strength and Conditioning Association's Personal Training Conference, which just happens to be my favorite conference of the year. I'm happy to say that, as usual, it did not disappoint. I had the opportunity to learn from some of the most successful fitness professionals in our field.

My favorite presentation was given by Shelby Murphy from *Personal Fitness Professional* magazine. Shelby presented various ways to improve client retention and to develop what we call "lifers". "Lifers" are clients who establish a wonderful, trusting and dedicated relationship with their trainer and, in turn, choose to continue their training sessions for life. Establishing a training schedule full of "lifers" is every personal trainer's dream. I have worked very hard over the last eleven years to develop my clientele to the point at which the majority of my schedule (about 90%) are "lifers." Shelby pointed out how these "lifers" can literally make a trainer hundreds of thousands of dollars over the time they train together. Between the consistent training schedule and the constant referrals, the "lifer" is a trainer's biggest fan.

My longest tenured "lifer" is Ruth Tesar. Ruth is a Masters downhill skier and has been training with me since 2004. Ruth was my first client, and has been training with me at least twice a week for the last seven years (I like to joke and say that Ruth has paid for both my Bachelor's and Master's degrees). After hearing Shelby talk about how a "lifer" can have such a positive long term financial impact, I decided to take a look back at my books and see exactly how much money Ruth has actually made me. I was shocked to find out that she literally has paid for both of those degrees! From one very grateful personal trainer to my longest tenured "lifer", I would like to say thank you, Ruth! Without you and all of your support, my career and the culture we have developed in our gym would not be where they are today. I hope all trainers have the opportunity and privilege to work with a "lifer" like Ruth. She truly is a pleasure to work with.

Shelby Murphy, Jay Dawes, Todd Miller, Loren Landow, Leo Totten and Jeremy Boone were all fantastic presenters at the conference, and I learned a great deal from all of them. Fitness (much like the internet) has grown into a social network in which education, program design, strategies and communication skills are shared from peer to peer. I must say that it is a very nice feeling to be accepted, even though only slightly at this point, into the fitness circle of trust. I am sure it will take me a few more years to gain their trust and to be fully accepted. That's the way it should be, and I'm more than happy to earn my stripes.

I also had the privilege of meeting many young personal trainers who are just starting out in their careers. They remind me of my experiences years ago when I was in their same position. Best of luck to all of you, and remember to be the absolute best you can be and never settle for anything less. It is not fair to you or your clients to do so.

The NSCA, as usual, delivered a wonderful product, and I am happy to say I'm coming home with some new tricks up my sleeve. Thank you to all the presenters who shared their information and experiences with us. Also, thank you to the NSCA for hosting such a great event. CPT Consultants, my private consulting business, made its first professional appearance at this conference. I have been privately mentoring certified personal trainers all across the country for the last ten years, and took my business public this past February. The conference was a great place to start; we had many trainers stop by and interact with us. I hope this is the beginning of something great as my passion for it grows every day.

Thank you to all of you who subscribe to this newsletter. Your funds are directly applied toward my continued education as I strive to obtain new information to write about in my newsletters and share with you. Thank you so much for all the support. Make today a great day. You should take one step toward achieving something you didn't think possible.

Americans vs. Europeans

Having participated in track and field (hammer throw) and weightlifting (clean & jerk/snatch), I have seen my share of European athletes. These sports are, for the most part, dominated by Europeans. I have noticed over the years that European athletes generally have very different body compositions than American athletes, and I think I have a pretty good idea why.

The American media has painted for us a picture of what we are "supposed" to look like in order to appear sexy or physically fit. Magazines, television and internet ads suggest that the "everyday female" is supposed to be as skinny as can be; that curves are no longer sexy, and big boobs and a tight ass are a must. This wrongful depiction of the American woman is what causes young ladies to turn to eating disorders like anorexia and bulimia, and to have breast enhancement surgery before they are even fully developed. The media-portrayed female image in America is so far from healthy, and it's too bad that it has developed to where it is today.

Men, on the other hand, are sold on big upper body muscles and a six pack. There was one point in my life in which I got to see my six pack, and it was only there for about a week. I was 6% body fat and had leaned out from 260 down to 192 pounds for an all-natural body building show. Some people, like me, will only see their six pack (which is actually an eight pack, but most people don't know that) in situations like this. Others are naturally gifted with high metabolisms, and will see their eight packs every day regardless of what they eat. This idealized image of the American male pushes young men into taking steroids to be able to achieve the standards of today's "muscular male body". Again, this exemplifies the American media pushing us toward something that is not healthy for us.

Europeans, on the other hand, aspire toward a different body image. Curves are considered sexy on women, and all body types, shapes and sizes are accepted. The European athlete has fantastic legs and a strong core, but not necessarily the best upper body. Americans like what we call "the mirror muscles", which are any muscles that you can see in the mirror when you face it. Americans like to do bench presses and biceps curls. Throw in a thousand sit-ups (to tighten up the hip flexors and hurt the back) and some quad extensions (to over develop the front of the thigh causing tight hamstrings and a hunch back) and we are good to go. By contrast, Europeans take value in the dead lift. They know how important it is to lift things up off the floor correctly.

Don't get me wrong; I'm not anti-America or anti-bench press by any means. However, I do think that the European mindset in regards to body image and fitness training is a much healthier, and makes setting fitness related goals a much more reasonable process. This is why I do not have any weight machines in my weight room. Every one of my clients learns how to dead lift properly, without the help of a machine. That is why every one of my clients learns to perform the Olympic lifts in some way, shape or form. And, that is why you will hear me say that hamstrings and lats are damn sexy muscles. I want everyone to have a healthy and reasonable body image. I want people to value their health and their body to the point where they pick up their shoes off the floor correctly rather than simply bending over quickly. Take pride in your body as you train it to be well-rounded. Don't forget the muscles on the back side - they are the most important in relation to proper posture and bone density longevity.

My message is this: please do not fall into the American media trap and believe that that is what we are "supposed" to look like. There is so much value in having a healthy figure with some meat on your hamstrings and being able to perform a proper chin up. This is only my opinion, as I have no scientific evidence to support my stance; however, this is the way I teach and it is the standard to which I consistently hold my clients. Every day they come into my gym to improve their bodies by training the all their bodies' muscles, not just the muscles they can see in the mirror. There is no negative self-talk allowed in my facility. We are a "good energy" gym, and feed off of the "good energy" from others. I hope you find some insight on this topic and make a change for the better. Remember, Roman dead lifts are sexy, sit-ups are not!

The Lower Case C

Remember the movie *Freaky Friday,* with Jamie Lee Curtis and Lindsay Lohan? There is a scene where they first switch bodies (mother and daughter, due to a Chinese magic spell) and Jamie realizes she is in her daughter's body. She makes a reference to her butt, saying her lower case "C" butt has become an upper case "C" over the years. This saying refers to the profile view of the butt; high and tight is a lower case "C". The only time I have heard this line used was in this movie until I recently started working with a new female client. During her assessment I asked her what her goals were. The first words out of her mouth were, "lower case C". Verbally, I was stuck for a second and didn't even know how to respond until it hit me and I understood what she was talking about.

The term "lower case C" has now become part of my vocabulary when I discuss training techniques with my female clients. After our initial assessment, my new client signed up for a personalized program design for which I created workouts for her to do on her own. The main goal of these workouts was to establish a foundation of strength around which we could develop her entire body. The second goal was to get her strong enough so that she could perform an exercise that would greatly increase her chances of developing that "lower case C" butt she wanted so badly. That exercise is called a Bulgarian Lunge in Place. I would like to discuss how to perform this specific exercise with all of you, just in case your "C" isn't where you want it to be.

Bulgarian Lunge in Place

In my opinion, this is the number one exercise for working the caboose. It is performed much like a lunge in place, but instead of keeping both feet on the ground, the rear leg is elevated anywhere from four to 12 inches. Elevating the rear foot increases the leg's range of motion. This increase specifically focuses on stretching the rear hip flexor. The primary mover in the exercise is the gluteus maximus (your butt!). The front leg's gluteus does the majority of the work.

We use the phrase "ski jump" to refer to the position in which the pelvis is un-tucked (tail bone sticking out). The lower back and the top of the butt invert to create a slope, or a ski jump. This is the premiere hip position for all lower body work (back squats, front squats, Roman dead lifts, step ups, lunges, etc.) and should be a constant coaching point for every certified personal trainer. If you want that "ski jump - lower case C" butt, make sure your tail bone is sticking out, lower back is arched, chest is up, shoulders are back, and both legs are performing the movement with equal effort (50/50). Many inexperienced fitness enthusiasts perform lunges and Bulgarians by loading the front leg. This can cause major knee issues, so please practice this move safely. If in doubt, ask a fitness professional.

Once the body weight Bulgarian Lunge in Place is mastered, you can increase your "C" by adding weight. I prefer the "Goblet" position. The Goblet position is performed by holding either a kettle bell or a dumbbell in front of the body with both hands. Imagine you are holding a large Goblet from the days of old and are preparing to take a drink from it. Holding the weight on the front of your body recruits your core to work harder than usual (I have often told my clients the best core work you can do is the front squat).

The Goblet position is similar to the front squat position, but without the extra pressure on the wrist. Using proper technique when performing the Goblet position can develop a very strong core and provide the "overload" that we are looking for to train that "lower case C." The term "overload" for a certified fitness professional is seen as a positive thing. Overloading the muscle places stress on the muscle to work hard and that is how it begins to grow and get stronger over time. When discussing an exercise with too much weight or too many repetitions, we use the term "excessive load".

Here is the primary message of this newsletter: utilize the Bulgarian Lunge in Place to increase the strength and size of your "C," but do so correctly. Too much of anything is bad for your body, so start off slowly.

Three sets of 12 repetitions on each leg will be more than enough to get you good and sore on the first day.

Remember, quality over quantity! Always! As you get stronger, don't be afraid to lift some heavier weight. As I have discussed in previous newsletters, building muscle burns more fat than anything else. Ditch the cardio and lift some weights to build the "C" you have always dreamed of.

Checking For Pain

The good thing about working with so many different people is that I am provided with varying topics and inspiration for my newsletters. Today's newsletter was inspired by a new client of mine who has some unique physical limitations. She severely rolled her ankle when she was young, and has had problems with it ever since. While talking to her about her injury, I noticed that she continued to push her knees forward in an attempt to stretch her ankle.

I asked her why she was performing that particular movement, and she answered by saying that it felt good to stretch the muscles in her ankle. I then informed her that the problem with this stretch is that she is repeatedly pushing her knees out beyond her toes. Even though this feels good at the moment, it causes long term damage to the knee. I work with many people with multiple physical limitations, and oftentimes I find they have developed similar habits of compensating for those limitations by performing potentially damaging stretches or exercises.

For example, rounding your back while standing feels fantastic on the lumbar, as this movement stretches the muscles in the lower back. Unfortunately, when standing, this places a lot of pressure on the lumbar vertebra. Performing this stretch while on the knees (downward dog or tiger stretch as we call it) allows for the same stretching without putting pressure on the lower back. Another example is holding the hands together and passing the arms all the way over head and behind the back. This movement shows great flexibility, but can also cause major damage if not done correctly. Clearly, there are many stretches that feel good but may not have a positive effect on our bodies. Now, we understand that static stretching may not be the best thing for our muscles in the first place.

An injury or physical limitation can also cause someone to incorrectly "test" the area in question. Someone who has a physical limitation or an acute (short duration of time) injury will often try to test the injured area by contracting it or moving in the specific range of motion that triggered the pain before, checking for pain each time the motion is performed. The problem here is that every time a person "checks" for pain, the injured area that was in the process of healing becomes re-injured again.

When you injury yourself, even mildly, you need to allow the injured area time to rest, recover and rebuild. By moving the injured area around, you are not allowing this process to take place. Do not "test" the injured area for at least 72 hours. Ice, ice and more ice! Never put heat on an injured area (as we've learned, it only makes things worse - heating pads, Bengay, tiger balm, icy hot, and bio freeze should all be used for loosening up an tight muscle and not for rehabilitating an injured one).

The point to consider is this: just because it feels good does not mean it is good for you. Think about the mechanics of your body prior to pushing limbs or joints into certain positions. The human body is an amazing thing; it will heal itself from almost any major issue on its own. Allow this process to take place. If you think you have severely injured yourself, please go to the emergency room rather than try to fix the problem yourself. Be smart and be safe rather than sorry. We don't often think much of the minor injuries, but they can potentially cause more damage by turning into a chronic (long term) injury as a result of incorrect healing.

What We Lose With Age

When I was in college working on my kinesiology degree, I took a class in which we discussed the five components of physical fitness: muscular strength, muscular endurance, cardiovascular endurance, body composition and flexibility. We learned that each of these components will begin to deteriorate as we age if we do not keep improving them. Have you heard the saying "use it or lose it?" It is usually implied when discussing muscle mass, but it is also relevant to each of these five fitness categories.

If you discontinue applying overload to your muscles (lifting weights), the muscles are no longer being used. As time goes on and the muscle is not called upon to work hard, it will begin to deteriorate. If you have ever broken a bone and had to wear a cast, this is why your limb looks small and frail after you get that cast off. Those muscles have not been used for a long period of time and have begun to atrophy (shrink).

The ratio of lean body mass (muscle, bone and organs) to fat is called body composition. If a body goes untrained for a long period of time, its metabolism, which begins to slow down as we age anyway, slows down even faster. Overeating causes a pile-up of unusable calories which are stored as fat. Body composition transfers as body fat increases. Weight training not only burns fat calories, but also boosts the metabolism at the same time. Interval training with weights causes your metabolism to work even harder and for a longer period of time even after your workout is completed. This is why weight training is the best way to increase lean muscle mass and decrease body fat as we age. Weight training not only helps us stay thin; it also helps us stay flexible if the exercises are performed correctly.

Muscles that are not trained in a full range of motion (FROM) will not stay flexible. I have written previously about the different types of stretching and which of those types are most beneficial. If you did not receive that email, please let me know and I will send you a copy. Weight training, when performed with the correct full range of motion and correct technique, has been proven to increase flexibility. Good flexibility is beneficial because flexible muscles assist in preventing injury. Spastic, stumbling movements like tripping over a curb or hopping two steps on the same foot until you eventually lose your balance and tumble down onto your side are less likely to produce an injury at age 20 when a person is more flexible than at age 70, when a fall like this would likely cause a broken hip, dislocated shoulder, or massive bruising to an untrained individual.

Old, inflexible, and weak muscles do not hold the bones together as do younger muscles. Catastrophes like broken bones can be avoided by weight training with correct technique in a full range of motion. I have 65+ year old clients who have informed me after a stumble that they would have been injured much worse had they not been training with weights for so many years. Instead of numerous broken bones, they come away with a small scratch and maybe a bruise or two.

Cardiovascular endurance is most important for keeping the organs in good working form. Well functioning organs are vital for living a long and healthy life. Most people believe that running on a treadmill, riding a bike, or pumping on a stair stepper (which just so happens to be the worst cardiovascular exercise you can perform) is the only way to increase cardiovascular endurance.

This is not the case. Interval training increases maximal heart rate and then allows it to recover multiple times during a single session. This is more beneficial for the heart and the lungs than 30 minutes at 65% maximal heart rate. The heart becomes used to that 65% tempo, whereas with interval training, the next level can always be accomplished by using more weight, performing more repetitions, and increasing the intensity of the interval exercise (jumping rope, rowing on the erg or running stairs).

My message is this: weight training with intervals will assist you in staying strong, keeping your muscles flexible, improving the working quality of your organs and improving your body composition. If there is a one-stop-shop in fitness, I would say you have found it. Machines have their place in fitness. They assist the injured or beginning weight trainer in developing a base level of strength, flexibility and endurance.

Once developed, this individual is ready for the next challenge. In my program design, I move those who have established this base level to pulleys. Pulleys allow for a freer range of motion, but also provide some control of the movement. Free weights are the next step, and are the ultimate goal for each of my clients. Free weights (dumb bells, bar bells and kettle bells) allow you to manipulate the weight however you like. This, when performed correctly, produces stable joints and strong, flexible and well-trained muscles.

Why My Back Hurts

I started weight training when I was 13 years old by working out with my sister's boyfriend at a gym in Zephyr Cove, Nevada. On my first day, I learned how to back squat. I remember feeling the pump in my legs after a set. I grew to love that feeling, and craved it every time I worked out. By the time I got to high school I was squatting over 250 pounds (I have to add that this was, by far, the best of anyone in our freshman class!). During my senior year, I joined the 500-pound club and earned a T-shirt from my coach. I was known for my squats, and had the best technique around.

Then I got to college, and found that front squatting was more applicable to throwing the hammer than back squatting, so I taught myself how to front squat. After a few years of doing it on my own, I started to feel some pain in my lower back. I did not have a weight room coach working with me every day; I trained on my own. I was "invincible" at that point in my life, and thought that nothing could hurt me. Slowly, my back kept getting worse and worse, and eventually it got to the point where I could no longer bend over to pick up my hammers. I would have to hook the handle with my foot and then bring it up to my hand. Regardless of how much pain I was having, I finished my junior year with x-rays that showed nothing wrong in my back.

Senior year came, and with it came a goal of front squatting 500 pounds. My best at that point was 395 pounds, so I knew I had some work to do. As the track and field season grew closer, my strength levels grew higher. I maxed out in front of the football team at 440 pounds (200 kilos), and was thrilled. I knew that with one or two more years of training, I would achieve my goal of 500. I finished the season with mild back pain, but nothing like what I was experiencing the previous year. I had backed off the front squats for a while, and that had seemed to help. I finished my senior season, and threw the next two years for Reebok. I retired in 2006 and started a career in all natural body building.

In 2008, I decided to return to throwing the hammer and started my year off right. New Years day, 6:00 a.m., my wife and I got to her gym bright and early. I put on my normal warm-up weight of 225. I squat down to parallel, and feel this massive rip and a shift in my lower back. Being as stubborn as I am, I didn't dump the bar; instead, I made myself stand up. This damaged my back even further. I could not straighten up all the way and eventually ended up on the floor. For 30 minutes I lay there, waiting for someone to help me. No one came and eventually I made myself get up. I walked up front and told my wife that I had hurt my back again and was going home to ice it. It was the longest and most painful car ride of my life.

Three nights of no sleep and a doctor's visit later I was home with some major pain killers and a packet of steroids to decrease the inflammation to my disc. My MRI showed two bulging discs and one rupture. At first my doctor thought he had the wrong images. He told me this couldn't possibly be my back. He then asked if I had been in a car accident. I told him my story, and eventually we traced it back to poor squatting technique in high school and college. My throwing career was over; my lifting career was over, my body building career...over. It took me some time but, eventually, I learned from this experience and took away a lesson from it that I now carry on to my clients and to all of you reading this. Technique is everything, which is why I harp on you all so much when you are training with me. Those who can no longer do, teach. I have learned from my mistakes and I do not want any of you to have to do the same.

I am famous for saying, "chest up and butt out." This is the position I never mastered. I had the "chest up" part down, but I never quite got the "butt out" part mastered. That is why my back was forced to hold all the weight I was squatting. I often say the back is like an electrical cord. You can bend it, twist it, squeeze it, and pull on it and nothing will happen until one day, without warning, it will snap. My message to you is this: I often preach that lifting heavy weight is good for you, but I want you to understand that you must master good technique prior to doing so. Lifting weights with poor technique is like riding on a motorcycle with no helmet. All it takes is one accident and you are toast. Please pay attention to your technique. If you think you are doing something wrong, please do not be embarrassed to ask for help. There is no shame in it.

A few months after my MRI, I had back surgery which released the pain in my back immediately. I did not have my back fixed; I simply had the painful rupture removed. If I start to lift incorrectly or too heavy, my back will begin to hurt again and that is never a good thing. Any of you who have thrown your back out know what I am talking about. It is the worst pain you have ever felt, and you can't do anything about it. Please take care of your back; it is the only one you get. There are no back replacements. Remember that the muscles in the lower back need to be trained to be strong. That old saying, "don't lift with your back" is wrong. It should instead be, "don't lift with poor technique." That is where the injury occurs.

Value your back and your body, and please understand that if you continue to do things wrong over and over again you will eventually pay the price. I hope you never have to experience any of the issues I have had to deal with, and that is why I am constantly on every one of my client's asses about proper technique. "It must be done correctly; don't end up like me," I tell them.

Get Off the Elliptical

It's a good idea - a machine that allows a person to replicate the form of running without impact. However, the design is awful. Machine trainers, like Cybex, Life Fitness, Free Motion, Precor and all other cardiovascular equipment are, in my opinion, for injured individuals who are trying to rehabilitate an injury or for beginners who are new to working out and need to build a basic foundation of strength. For the avid fitness enthusiast or athlete, I strongly suggest you stay far away from these machines. The problem starts with a person's "gait."

A "gait" is the dimensions of a person's naturally occurring walking or running stride. For example, I'm six-foot three inches and I have a 30-inch walking and a 44-inch running gait. Compare me to a four-foot nine inch gymnast who has a 20-inch walking and a 32-inch running gait. Should the two of us exercise on the same elliptical? No; it would restrict my gait and increase hers. That is why the elliptical is not good for any healthy individual. I'm sure there is the perfect sized person out there who matches up well with that machine, but we don't know what height or what gait fits it correctly.

The next time you are in the gym, stand behind someone on the elliptical and watch their knees, hips and shoulders. We have a few "Stevie Wonders" at our gym. They place their hands so high up on the elliptical handles that they literally weave from side to side the way Stevie does when he is singing. The knees buckle in toward each other and cross the mid-line (the line right down the middle of your body, facing front) or they bow out like they just got off a horse.

Both of these knee displacements are caused by the gait not matching the person's who is using the machine. The hips will often pop from side to side as well, or will stick out slightly. This occurs when the person forces their legs and gait to match the elliptical. The only way they can do that is by sticking their butt out and shortening their stride, which is what happens to people who have a gait that is too long for the elliptical.

I started this newsletter by saying the elliptical is a good idea but a bad design. I wish I knew how to design a better one, but that is not my area of expertise. So what about all you folks out there who need low- or no-impact training? Get in the pool! There is no impact in the pool or very little depending on what exercises you are performing. Try treading water for 30 minutes and see how tired you are after that. I got up to 60 minutes once after my back surgery. Yes, it's a little boring, so investing in a water proof iPod may be a good idea. How about the rowing machine? No impact there. The recumbent bike? Not the best thing because you are sitting down.

People sit down all day long, that is where the majority of us spend our days. We sit...at work...all day long. Then we go to the gym and do the same thing. Let me tell you this: if you are reading the newspaper and doing your "cardio" (I hate this word) at the same time, you are not working hard enough. I ride the recumbent bike two to three times per week because of my low back and I work hard on that puppy. No way could I sit and read at the same time. Watch "The Bachelor", yes. Read *USA Today,* no.

Why do I hate the word "cardio?" Because it is an overused word that generally describes people walking, running or biking on machines at 60% of their maximal heart rate for 30 to 60 minutes. Is this going to help you make improvements to your body? No, at least not very much. If you are recovering from a disease, like cancer, then the "cardio" machines are the place to start, but your goal should be to get off them as soon as possible. "Cardio" machines have their place. I used to walk for 60 minutes every morning for the first six months after my lung cancer surgery. That is what I needed then and now that I am able to do more, I interval train.

Alwyn Cosgrove, in his book *The New Rules of Lifting,* discusses the results of two exercise groups. One group performs 60 minutes of cardiovascular exercise on a treadmill or elliptical for four weeks and burns a certain amount of calories. Another group performs 30 minutes of interval weight training for three weeks and burns half as many calories but loses NINE times as much fat. Burning calories does not always mean burning fat. In this case, the elliptical group is burning more muscle than fat. The interval group is building muscle, which, in turn, burns more fat at the same time. As Alwyn would say, "The captain has turned off the 'cardio' light; please feel free to move about the weight room!"

There are two things I want you to get from my newsletters: passion and education. I study this stuff all the time, and I would not be as passionate about it if I didn't know that it was true. Join the fitness revolution today and stop wasting your time on the elliptical. Or, start tomorrow if you like. The fitness revolution can begin at any time. Stop doing the same old things that have given you the same old results. It's time for something new! If you have physical limitations, we can work around them. If you think you are too old, you are not. If you think you won't succeed, you are wrong. All you need is the right team behind you and a support group around you. Find this in your life, and you will accomplish your fitness goals.

I Don't Have Time

I am guiltier than any of you of this one. I get so consumed in my work or with my hobbies (writing newsletters!) that I don't allow myself enough time in the day to exercise. My father once told me, "If something is important to you, you will make time for it no matter what." This is the mindset we should maintain when scheduling exercise into our daily routines. We all know that exercising is good for us, yet we still allow it to be the first thing we cut from our day if we get behind. We allow our jobs to take priority over the one thing that can prolong our lives, make us feel better and improve our quality of life. I had an appointment today with a brand new client, and during that assessment session he told me how much better he felt after starting his workout routine. He has been performing a basic circuit routine around the weight room for the last four months and is now ready for the next step. That next step brought him to me.

He was very sincere when he said he felt better after starting his program. I think a lot of us don't really recognize how great we do feel when we finish a solid workout. Yes, we are tired and sweaty. However, deep down inside, we feel energized and awake. We experience something called a "lifter's high" for the next few hours. What is the lifter's high? Same thing as a "runner's high", except without the running. The endorphins and hormones in your body are running high, which in turn creates a sense of euphoria or, in some cases, nausea until the body gets used to working that hard. Your metabolism will be burning on high for the next few days after training with weights. This combined with a healthy diet will result in fat loss, stronger muscles, and a more endured cardio-respiratory system.

Please think about these great qualities, and start to value them for so much more than what they really are. Maintaining a healthy body is such an important part of our lives, and in order to do so we must exercise often. I'm right there with some of you; I am guilty of not doing my workout every day because I'm tired or have too much work to do. If it is important to me, I will find the time to do it. I have not placed as much value on my quality of life since I regained my health. I dove right into work rather than focusing on improving my body.

Please learn a lesson from me and take my word for it - you don't want to head down this road. Make a change for the better. The nice thing about exercise is that it is never too late to start getting in shape.

For some of us, our workout will be walking on a treadmill until we are healthy enough to increase intensity and move to the next step. Others will need a seven-days-a-week program to see results. This is where a professional like me comes in handy. If you need assistance learning where you should begin, just let me know. I want you all to value your health and not to take it for granted, I did once, and I almost lost it. Take a step toward improving yourself every day. It's never too late to start. I'm here with you! You have a team behind you! Now it's up to you to take that first step and join the fitness revolution. Do not conform to the old way of exercising. Educate yourself on the right way to get fit. Education is the key to success and that is, "The Fitness Revolution!"

Beauty and the Bench Press

I want you to take a moment and remember the last time you laid on your back and pushed something directly off your chest. Other than bench pressing your kids in bed on a Sunday morning, can you think of anything else? I write often about something called "functional training". Functional training means that the exercises you perform are assisting you in building strength for your everyday movements.

For example, I train a businessman who constantly has to carry a 15 to 20 pound briefcase wherever he goes. During his training, we do one arm farmer walks to balance his body. This "functional" exercise is not only making him stronger for carrying his briefcase; it is also balancing his imbalance from always carrying it on the same side. Since we started working together, he rotates his briefcase from side to side often.

When it comes to the bench press, I can't really see any functional movement relevance. Maybe for MMA fighting, when you are trying to get someone off of you? Not sure; I don't follow that sport much. Offensive linemen (football) are standing when they are pushing on people, so performing a "jammer" or "Neider press" is much more functional (push press type exercise at a 45 degree angle). If it's not functional, then why are we, as fitness enthusiasts, so obsessed with it? If one guy asks another guy if he works out and that guy says yes, there is a 99 percent chance that the next question will be, "How much do you bench?" Is this a form of judgment? Do we now have gym cliques, those who bench and those who don't? Don't get me wrong, I like to bench and work it into my routine every other week or so. However, I use it to assist me in improving my push-up strength.

Push-ups, on the other hand, are a very functional movement. We are getting up off the floor often with our kids, in sporting events, and in our regular lives. Pushing yourself out of bed in the morning resembles a push-up more than any other movement. The strength you build from push-ups is a strength that I feel all of my clients need in their daily lives, and that is why we perform push-ups almost daily. It is a movement that we need to be able to perform efficiently. Although bench pressing has less functional importance than do push-ups, it's still okay to incorporate it into your workout routine. Work it in as you like into your personal programs, but understand why you are performing it.

Squats are another functional movement that we perform more than any other movement on a daily basis. Getting into the car, standing up from a desk, getting up off the couch, or standing up from a chair are all forms of a squat. We squat constantly, and that is why there is ALWAYS a squat in every workout I perform, write or coach. My message to you is this: remember the real reason for working out. We need to grow strong enough to perform daily life movements and to prevent injury upon entering an odd movement or asking the body to respond to a stimulus quickly.

You won't believe the number of "I grabbed my kid before he or she got hurt and ended up hurting myself," stories I have heard. Throwing out your back bending over to grab the baby, tweaking your neck after your daughter jumped on your back or having the dog hyper-extend your knee are all issues that I help my clients deal with on a daily basis. I want you to be functional enough that when these things happen you get through them injury free.

Full body strength is a must, and is what the "Fitness Revolution" is all about. Please, if you currently do this, get away from the "split" body routine. The "split" body routine entails working the chest and triceps one day, back and biceps the next, shoulders and abs the following day, and legs on the last day. The Fitness Revolution (thanks to the NSCA) has proven that training the entire body on a daily basis is the most "functional" and the most efficient way to change your body's composition (lose fat and gain muscle).

Sorry to all you body builders out there (I used to be one of you). In my opinion, the "split" routine is dead. It's time for a change, and training the entire body in functional movements is just what the doctor ordered. Remember this: you are all regular people before you are anything else. Take the appropriate steps to ensure your body will stay as healthy as possible as you get older.

Take it from me; I thought I was indestructible for a very long time until, one day, I broke. Nothing hurts your ego more than finding out you were wrong. I want to spare you some of this pain so please, please, please: take the appropriate steps toward instilling a healthy future. Functional movements that are technically sound are so much better for the body than heavy weight with poor technique. I know there are some out there who will disagree with me, and that is okay.

I would rather slightly under-train my clients so they can always train than over train my clients once and have them get injured. I have done this in the past (five years ago) and trust me, it sucks to be the trainer responsible for injuring someone permanently. I know that I have matured and educated myself since this incident, and I deeply believe that what I do now is the best thing for all my clients and for all of you reading this newsletter. I hope you all stay healthy and functional. Be smart, train smart and stay the course. Tomorrow brings another opportunity to improve yourself!

Farmers and Waiters and Walks...Oh My!

You have just returned from the grocery store and you are getting ready to carry in all those grocery bags. Instead of taking two at a time, you decide to carry three or four bags on each arm (which crushes the bread by the way) to save time. You have to walk from the car and up the drive way, through the garage, through the living room and finally into the kitchen. As you set the bags down, you realize you are breathing heavy and that the muscles in your arms are spent. Does this sound like something you have done before? This is called a "farmer's walk," and it is one of my favorite exercises.

The exercise is simple: carry weight on both sides or on one side while maintaining a tight core with your tail bone tipped out, keeping your elbows slightly flexed and keeping a tiny shrug in your shoulders just to protect the joints. My instructions include a technical talk about walking as well. Pretend you have to go to the bathroom really badly. Any kind of bouncing up and down will only make the urge to go worse. This same concept applies to the farmer's walk. If big steps are taken, the body will slightly bounce up and down.

This will create momentum that will cause the weights to bounce, and the elbow and shoulder joints are not as stable as they should be if the weights are bouncing. Short, steady and smooth flowing steps are required to provide a solid core, no bouncing, and a fast and efficient movement (no pun intended). Try carrying 30 pound dumbbells from one end of the weight room and back three times, or pick up two kettle bells and walk around the basketball court. Not only are you improving your core strength, but your grip strength as well.

How about the "waiter walk"? Instead of holding the weights down at your sides (farmer walk), try holding them up, the way a waiter would hold a tray, to the side of your head. The elbow should be flexed to 90 degrees and should be actively holding the weight (actively meaning do not allow the weight to rest on the biceps or on the shoulders; actively hold the weight up at that 90 degree angle and proceed with walking). Want to make it harder? Try holding two (one in each hand) and walk up and down stairs (be careful!).

Try to hit every other step on the way up and every step on the way down. This exercise starts off very easy but gets hard in a hurry. Remember why you are performing this exercise. You are focusing on producing proper posture and developing great core strength. Once your posture starts to break down and you can no longer hold it correctly, stop the walk and rest for a bit. Your training should always be based on proper technique and not on how much, how many, or how fast you can perform.

My last newsletter discussed the functional application of the bench press to real life. This exercise (farmer's walk/waiter's walk) replicates and trains the body for movements we perform all the time. That is why they have the names that they do. Farmers are notorious for carrying buckets of feed, fertilizer or seed out to a specific location. Oftentimes that location is a ways away. Because of this, farmers developed fantastic core and grip strength from carrying these heavy buckets or tools to these far off destinations. As far as functional application is concerned, it doesn't get more functional than this. We do this movement often; however, we normally perform it on one side.

Think about carrying your kids, your briefcase, your purse, a travel bag, a gallon of paint, or whatever you might be carrying. Do you hold it, or them, with both hands evenly in front of your body with perfect posture and a tight core, with your butt slightly out while taking small steps? Not usually. So if you can train yourself to carry a 25 pound dumbbell in your right hand, walk 75 meters, switch hands and walk back, then you can develop the core strength necessary to carry your eight pound purse or 12 pound briefcase around all day with proper posture and with no trouble at all.

This movement is very functional, and can be beneficial for all of us. At one point or another we are slightly or heavily overloaded on one side of our bodies. Training the body to be prepared for this movement will not only make you successful at it, but assist you in preventing injury as well. I had a client tell me yesterday that he wants to prolong his quality of life as long as possible. In my mind that means preventing injury or sickness, and those are two areas in which I feel very good about helping my clients improve. If you can train your body to be healthy and free of injury, I believe you will have a great quality of life in the long run. One thing about fitness: you are never going to be too strong or too fit. Fitness is a never ending cycle, and I want you to always be able to keep up with or get slightly ahead of that cycle.

Keep your body strong for as long as possible so you can simultaneously prolong a high quality of life. I have seen 75 year-old fitness enthusiasts who look like they're 55 because they have taken such good care of their bodies. I have also seen 40 year-olds who look like they're 60 because they haven't taken good care of themselves. The old saying "we are what we eat" applies to the fitness level of the body as well. Your body will reflect the amount of work you put into it.

If you work hard, your body will also be hard and will last a long time. If your work ethic is soft, then your body will be soft and will slowly begin to break down. Be proactive; it is never too late to make a change. Please do not take your quality of life for granted. Instead, cherish it! Work hard for it! And never let it leave your area of focus, as this is the one thing in life that will keep you in good spirits.

Power of the Plank

The contraction of a muscle or muscles without movement is called isometric training, and it is utilized to perform one of the simplest exercises to train the core. The plank looks easy enough to perform. However, it requires more effort from the core muscles to hold the body in perfect alignment for one minute than it does to perform 30 sit-ups. On a quick side note: I have said this privately to many of my clients in the past and have hinted at it in a few of my newsletters, but I now feel confident in saying to all of you now - SIT UPS ARE BAD FOR YOU! Please stop doing them! Types of sit-ups include leg lifts, Russian twists, V-ups, and crunches, and the one that is particularly bad for you is the decline sit up bench.

I know what some of you are saying: "We just did Russian twists and V-ups a month ago in my class." This is true. However, I have learned from some of the brightest professionals in the fitness industry that these positions, when performed incorrectly, can be devastating to the lower back. The real question is, on average, how many repetitions does it take to perform these two exercises incorrectly? In my experience, it only takes five to 10 repetitions. After five repetitions, the core muscles and hip flexors are not working efficiently enough to hold the lower back in the correct position. This in turn causes lower back pain.

So what should we include in our workout routines to emphasize core strength? The answer is the plank, or any variation of the plank. You can develop tremendous core strength by performing this exercise correctly. Let's start by looking at the proper posture of the exercise.

Take a second and please do the following: stand up and place your feet shoulder width apart. Stand tall with your shoulders back, chest up and head high. Now slightly (just an inch or two) unlock your hips (stick your butt out) and squeeze your abs tight (like someone is getting ready to sucker punch you, tighten up!). Keep a little bend in your knees and raise your arms out in front of you like a zombie. Keep the elbows where they are, and rotate your hands so your thumbs are up. Bend your elbows to 90 degrees, and make a fist. Now hold that position as tight as possible. This is your perfect posture plank position.

To perform a perfect plank, you need to be able to put yourself in that position while laying face down on the floor.

The key to the plank is to keep your hips unlocked (butt sticking out). There are many books and videos that state the back must be perfectly flat when performing the plank. This is not the case. Take it from a guy with a bad back; this is the right way to do it. Your butt should be sticking up just high enough to be level with your shoulders. I always tell my clients that they should be able to place their cup of coffee on their tail bone and not have it tip over. When you tuck your butt underneath you, all the pressure of your body sits on your spine (lumbar) rather than being supported by the core muscles.

When I say "stick your butt out," I don't mean raise your hips. This is what most of my clients do the first 30 times I correct them; I say butt up and they turn themselves into a tee pee. I want them to be able to keep the shoulders and the hips level and simply unlock or tilt the pelvic bone outwards. You can practice this movement by standing up tall and pulling your pelvis underneath you. Look at your lower back in the mirror as you do this. Without moving your hips forward or backward, tilt your pelvis outward so that your tailbone is now sticking out. Your lower back should make what we call the "ski jump" position. You want your lower back to arch outward and "ski jump" off your tailbone. Once you have mastered this movement standing up, you can then proceed to the floor and implement your "ski jump" during the plank. Do not practice the pelvic tilt too many times in the plank position because you can injure yourself by doing so.

Think of it in these terms: if you put both ends of an eight foot long 2x4 on cinder blocks, where is the weakest point of the board? Right - the middle. Now, place another cinder block right in the middle of the board. The middle is no longer the weakest point of the board. Place your elbows at one end and your toes at the other, where is the weakest point of your body? Yup, you guessed it - in the middle. If you can support the middle by hoisting it up (with your core), then you will continue to build strength in a perfectly postured position.

After reading this newsletter to my wife, she remarked that when she does her planks just as I ask, she cannot perform it as long as she normally can. That is because she is not strong enough to hold the plank in the correct position for that long of a period. This is where she needs to be honest with herself. All of us have a little bit of an ego (some more some less) when it comes to performing. We want to go as long as possible and push ourselves to get in better shape. The problem comes when the proper form is no longer being performed. The timer keeps ticking but the body is no longer improving. You have heard that old saying "practice makes perfect." This saying is wrong, it should read "perfect practice makes perfect."

My message to you is this: to improve core strength, the body must be in perfect balance in the perfect position. I have heard of a woman who performed a plank for 60 minutes once during a physical assessment test. Was she in the perfect position the entire time? I wasn't there so I can't say for sure, but I would guess that she was not. The effort required to hold a plank in perfect posture for two minutes is huge. Try maxing out your perfect posture plank and see how long you can last. Do this with a partner and have him watch your body. If you start to fold or break, have him call the time. If you don't trust his feedback, video tape it so you can see for yourself what you are doing wrong.

When you are testing your core strength, you cannot move your body at all. Once you are in place, you need to be like stone. As soon as you start to shift from side to side or lift one hand off the floor and shake it out, you have lost the true test of the core strength. The legs and shoulders have now come into play. This is a core strength test, not a full body test. Give it a shot and see how long you can make it. I will give you a goal. My best ever was 3:11. I did do a 5:15 once, but I did not have perfect technique. Shoot to beat my time, and I would love to hear about it when you do. Give me your feedback and let me know what you think.

I want you all to know that I appreciate you reading my newsletters. I hope that the information I provide for you helps you to improve your body and keeps you from getting injured. I am very passionate about my profession, and take it very seriously. If you need any questions answered, please do not hesitate to ask.

Please train smart and keep your body in good working order. I wish only great training for you all. Remember to push yourself every time you exercise, but do it with proper technique. Working within yourself and knowing your body well will give you a massive advantage, as you will continue to improve with every workout.

Chop That Wood

Science has recently shown us that one of the, if not the most efficient movements the human body can perform is splitting wood. I'm not talking about using a log splitting machine; I am referring to splitting wood the old fashioned way with an ax. The muscular effort required to raise an eight to 12 pound ax over head and the power required to pull down on the handle and deliver a blow powerful enough to split the wood in two is monumental. Repeating this movement over and over again while alternating the side with which you swing the handle will help you to become very powerful and balanced.

As cool as this would be, we do not have axes on the walls to use and wood laying around to split in the weightroom. Instead, we use a large medicine ball called a dynamax ball (DB). The DB is made of leather and is filled with layers of plastic wrapped with stuffing to give it the desired density. We take this ball over head and, utilizing the inertia from the hips, create downward velocity toward the floor and slam it to the ground with both hands. This replicates the wood chopping exercise rather well.

One way to improve your performance on a particular exercise is to work on the movement in reverse. Instead of swinging weight from over head down to the floor, we swing weight from between the knees up over head. We call this a "kettle bell swing." A kettle bell was made famous by some Russian muscle men who molded a kettle bell out of cast iron. The large handles and awkward weight distribution of the kettle bell made exercising with it a well rounded experience. Not only can you improve your strength by using the kettle bell, but also your balance, coordination and grip strength as well.

Looking at the wood chopping movement in reverse will give you a good understanding of how to perform a kettle bell swing. The swing, as simple as it looks, is a very technical exercise and should only be performed in the presence of a fitness professional until the skill is mastered. When we swing a kettle bell, we are working on the eccentric (lengthening) stretch of the muscles in the hamstrings and lower back.

As these muscles repeatedly perform eccentric stretches, they will continue to grow in strength. These muscles are the primary support muscles used to perform the wood chop exercise and are required to be strong if the exercise is to be repeated over and over. These muscles are also called "posture muscles" which are required to contract any time we are standing. There is a major correlation between developing these muscles while swinging a kettle bell and improving posture.

Yes, it looks a little crazy when you see it, but the benefits are so great enough that as long as you are healthy enough, you should start kettle bell swinging in your regular exercise routine. Again, this is a technique that takes time to learn and usually enters a program design (for beginners) after three months of basic strength building exercises. After about three months, the body is strong enough to handle this movement.

So if you are ever near my father-in-law's house and you feel like coming out and splitting some wood, just let me know and we can get you in for a good workout. In the past, Mike (my father-in-law) and I would head out to split wood early in the morning when the temperature was still down in the mid 30s. After five minutes or so of splitting wood, we were both down to our t-shirts and sweat pants having stripped off all our warm layers. This exercise is a workout all in its own, and I hope you get the opportunity to try it someday. Stay the course and thank you for joining the fitness revolution.

The Mind...is a Terrible Thing to Waste

On a daily basis at least one of my clients will come in for a workout all worked up about something that is happening in his or her life right at that moment. This could be the spouse not helping out, the kids are driving them crazy, an upcoming large dinner party, problems at work, heading off on vacation, starting a new business, tax season, the in laws are visiting, and many more. Trust me, I have heard them all. These are all legitimate issues that can produce a large amount of stress and in turn be detrimental to the overall health of the human body.

This stress is carried over into the workout and is distracting. I see it every workout; I'll provide instructions for the workout, demonstrate the exercises, provide instruction while demonstrating the exercise, and then ask if everyone understands or has a question (all heads seem to be listening and confirm understanding). I ask them all to get into position and instruct them all to begin. Nine out of 10 times I get at least one person who looks at me confused and says, "Wait, what are we doing?"

As a teacher (coach, instructor and trainer) this drives me crazy. I do understand that my loving clients are not doing this on purpose and have a lot on their minds. Exercise can be a fantastic way to reduce stress, but if the participants continue to stew over the stress while exercising, they cannot achieve its benefits.

This brings us to the purpose of this newsletter. I have a technique I would like you all to try next time you are stressed out prior to a workout. I have the added benefit of training all my clients in a private studio that allows this technique to work a little bit more effectively; however, it can work in any training facility or gym.

Prior to exercising, I want you to take a full 60 seconds in a space that is quiet. Go into the bathroom, sit in your car or stand in the corner. Close your eyes and repeat to yourself, "The next 60 minutes are for me and for me alone." Put all your other issues, stressors or problems aside for one hour and allow your mind to "relax" (yes, I said relax) while you are exercising.

This is easier said than done, I understand that, but this is the mindset that you need to focus on to allow this to work for you. If you can be mentally strong enough to allow you mind to relax and simply focus on the next 60 minutes of exercise you will feel much better afterwards. You mind will be at ease, your metabolism will be running high, you will have elevated endorphin levels that will bring that "euphoria" sensation (the lifters high – if you are a long time newsletter follower) and your energy levels will be boosted.

This hour does more for you than simply burn calories. This may be the only hour of the day that you have to be away from all the other things going on in your life. Take advantage of this opportunity. I often tell my clients to "put it aside and focus" when I can tell their minds are somewhere else. We need this time to step out of reality for a little while and allow the body to experience something great. Once you master this technique while exercising, you can begin to "relax your mind" while participating in other things as well (golf, tennis, swimming, etc.)

I do this prior to writing every one of these newsletters. I take a moment to settle my mind and focus my thoughts. I find that when I am writing, I'm not thinking about anything else. Once I complete my newsletter I feel that, for lack of better words, I come back to reality. Taking this small break from reality every few days leaves me feeling refreshed. It may sound goofy, but this can work for you if you believe in it. I want you to enjoy your workouts and to be "in the moment" when you are pushing yourself to new limits. Bring good energy with you as often as possible, as it will feed that "euphoria" feeling and leave you feeling balanced and fresh.

What We Don't Know Is Hurting Us

Late Monday afternoon, I flew down to Las Vegas for the 2nd Annual TSAC (Tactical Strength and Conditioning) Conference where 349 Army, Air Force, Navy, Marines, SWAT, Police, Sheriff, Fire Department, EMT, National Guard and any other people in national service came together to learn from some of the best and brightest in the business. I was the only "civilian" in the facility.

At least it felt that way. Everywhere I looked, I saw flat tops, shaved heads, perfect posture, muscles and intensity. I fit right in due to my receding hairline and posture (due to my back injury), so no one really questioned my being an outsider. But I was, and I had successfully infiltrated the facility to learn their secret ways. I have to admit, it was pretty awesome.

One of the presenters, Travis Harvey, PhD CSCS (Director of Human Performance for the 75th Ranger Regiment in Fort Benning, Georgia) had some very interesting information. He discussed the use of the "gravitron," or as some of us may know it, the "assisted pull up/dip machine." He and some associates wanted to learn the most efficient way to increase muscular strength in order to perform pull ups. Part of his job is to assist in training new recruits, and pull ups are a major part of their training. However, if they have someone who cannot perform pull ups, they want to know what would be the "best bang for their buck," so to speak. Through a series of tests, he made interesting discoveries.

To perform the pull up movements, our muscles have to contract in a certain sequence to manipulate the body into position. For example, when performing a pull up from the hanging position, the latissimus dorsi (lats) contract first, followed by the rhomboids, then the pectorals, and then the biceps. Harvey's discovery showed that on the gravitron machine, that sequence of muscular contractions was inverted. His information showed that using the gravitron to develop the strength to perform pull ups was actually the opposite of what is required to do one correctly. This information is shocking to the general fitness enthusiast because these machines are in practically every gym across the country.

This evidence shows that the gravitron will not assist in developing pull up strength nearly as efficiently as a jumping negative pull up will. A jumping negative entails gripping the bar with a slight bend in the elbows and being elevated enough to be able to use your legs to push your chin above the bar. From there, the body should be lowered down slowly. This is the "negative" part of the movement. A bunch of negatives will eventually equal a positive. With the feet free to move (unlike the gravitron, which has a step for the feet to stand on), the core muscles are being worked at the same time. This replicates a real chin up or pull up, and assists in developing the required amount of strength.

Sometimes, the machines or exercises we think are best for us actually our performances. Don't get me started on all the talks we had about not doing sit-ups. I love it! Every presenter touched on it at least once. There is a lot of evidence out there that proves, without a doubt, that sit-ups cause pain to the lower back, but that doesn't stop trainers and coaches alike from including sit-ups in their workouts.

Never again will I ever ask a client of mine to perform a sit-up (unless it's the first part of a Turkish-get-up)! I am sad to see other professionals in my business not take this information more seriously. It seems as if there is a fear of "changing the routine" that lurks in every personal trainer. They want to make workouts hard for their clients, not have them perform the most effective exercises.

I used to think that if I used the information that I just learned from a recent conference, my clients would think I was not intelligent and that I had simply implemented exercises invented by someone else. Honestly, I did! There are no new exercises to invent. Everything that I learn now is something that I have not seen or learned how to do yet. However, it's not a "new "exercise; it's just new to me. So, yes, I did take it from someone else and implement it into my program design.

But, I have to be smart enough to know how to use it, when to implement it into the program, how many repetitions to perform, and how much weight to lift. I have to be smart enough to teach the technique correctly and in the right order. This is not something you can learn over a weekend. This type of training comes from years of education in college, experience with clients, and earning certifications.

For all you certified personal trainers out there, please, please, *please* look at the research and advance your knowledge as our profession develops. We have some extremely intelligent, brilliant, even, individuals researching all of our training techniques. Read or allow yourself to be taught this information, and take it back to your clients to help them achieve something. Do not "just make 'em sweat;" we have already talked about that. It doesn't help; it only hinders.

For all you clients or fitness enthusiasts out there, do not follow blindly or do as others do without understanding why you are performing a certain exercise. Ask your trainer why you are performing the instructed exercises. If he or she can't answer you, RUN! This is not someone with whom you want to work. You need a passionate, intelligent and dedicated individual to work with who will take care of your body as if it were his own. That is the kind of person with whom you know you are in good hands. You only get one body; please take care of it. Think for yourself, be a student of fitness and learn how to exercise correctly. That is what the Fitness Revolution is all about.

It Looks Simple Enough

A couple of days ago I had two of my favorite clients working with the battle ropes. When I demonstrated the exercise, one of them said to me, "That looks simple enough." I smiled and said, "Good luck with that." These have been the humorous last words coming from many of my overly confident clients prior to me handing them their hat. After three rounds of swings, slams, slides, switch slams, and jump slams, this client was whistling to a different tune. When we got done he said it again: "Man... that *looked* simple enough," in an exhausted, half-hearted voice. "Why was that so difficult?"

In many cases, it's not the exercise that dictates the difficulty of the effort put forth. Program design is the primary reason behind a successful and challenging workout routine. What I mean by that is that selecting the appropriate weight for the appropriate amount of time or repetitions (volume) is most important than what exercises are included in a program. Any trainer can smash their clients into the ground by wrecking them in a workout. It takes a precise program design and progression to challenge a client just right. Take this routine for example. I would like you to perform 50 chin ups, 100 pushups and 150 squats all in a row before moving on to the next exercise. Do you think you could do that?

Some of you probably could; however, there are some of you who may not be able to complete the routine. What if I asked you to perform five chin ups, 10 pushups and 15 squats? Could you do that? Now repeat that round of exercises 10 times. This goal is much more attainable than trying to do all 50 chin ups in a row and so forth. It's all in the design. Just like training a new puppy not to go to the bathroom in the house, you need to set up your clients for success. If the program design in too hard, then the client performing the workouts will become discouraged. When a new client is done with a workout, I want her to feel fantastic. Exhausted, but fantastic. This will set up the rest of her day positively, as she has already started it off in the right direction. Now, insert impossible workout "name" here and make your client throw up afterwards. The day is now ruined.

Looking at an impossible workout to complete becomes overwhelming. I used to write these near-impossible and ridiculous workouts because I liked pushing my clients to the edge. My clients started to have little nervous breakdowns before our sessions because they would worry about how hard they were going to be. This is no longer the case, as my program design has improved. I now offer a much better product that is showing my clients great results. I have found that it's not about how hard I push my clients; it's about how well they perform when I ask them to push themselves. I would rather have clients push hard with perfect technique for 10 minutes than have them work with poor technique for 30.

My message to you is this: as a personal trainer, be smart about what you are prescribing to your clients. If you over train them, they will not be able to improve due to injury. You have now lost a client who is unhappy with the results you brought them. Instead, slightly under-train your clients, but train them consistently. Slow, consistent improvements add up over time and keep clients motivated, excited about training, and pumped because they are improving.

As the client, place trust in your trainer, as he or she should know what is best for you. If you feel like you are banged up all the time and exhausted from the workouts, then you may want to look for another line of exercise. If you are consistently improving, injury free, and are accomplishing your goals, then you are definitely with the right person. Commit yourself fully to that person and trust that what they are asking you to do will help you to reach your fitness goals.

Some workouts look easy written out on the board or while we, the trainers, are demonstrating a couple of reps. Believe that your trainer has a massive amount of education and experience, and they have everything you do programmed down to a T. As long as your trainer has proven herself to you, trust her 100 percent. If you are in doubt, find someone else, because every day wasted is another day lost toward getting into the best shape of your life.

There is more to improving yourself than engaging in a fad diet and a new bicep curl routine. It's a lifestyle change. That is what we (the proven certified personal trainers) are teaching you every single day. If you need help, if you have questions, if you need support, just ask. This is our job, and we love it! Commit to yourself and commit to your trainer and get yourself moving in the right direction. Stop waiting until tomorrow. As Apollo said in *Rocky III*, "There is no tomorrow! There is no tomorrow!"

Suspension Training: Just Hanging Around

It is a priceless look to capture when I bring new clients into our training studio and show them around. With eyes wide and the thoughts of, "What did I just get myself into," running through their heads, they focus in on the Olympic Rings (OR) or the Jungle Gyms (JG). Both of these devices are considered "suspension training" apparatuses and are a very integral tool in our style of training.

Pound for pound, the strongest athletes in the world are gymnasts. Gymnastics requires the perfect combination of conditioning, power, strength, balance, reaction time, coordination and flexibility to be successful in this sport. We, as trainers, have learned a thing or two from gymnasts over the years. The effort and body-awareness necessary to perform on the uneven bars or on the pummel horse is extremely high. The OR, in this regard, are no different. The OR are a very technical event and require years of practice and strength development to be able to safely perform on them. Where the average fitness enthusiast can benefit from the OR is in the many variations of training techniques that an educated certified personal trainer can teach you.

There are many variations including, but not limited to: the two handed or one handed reclined row, the two hand or one handed inverted row, ring roll outs, ring pushups, aviators, halos, dips, vertical pikes, pike ups and more. These exercises all share one major area of emphasis – core strength development. I have written in the past of the recent research supporting the argument that lumbar flexion exercises, like sit-ups and v-ups, cause damage to the lower back. I am often asked, "If sit-ups are no longer an option, how else can a fitness enthusiast work the core muscles?" I often answer with planks and plank variations, weighted holds including farm and waiter walks, and by working on the OR.

Much like the plank, the rings utilize the core to maintain the skeletal system in the proper posture during movement. Let's take a look at the ring roll out as an example. With the rings hanging from a pull-up bar above you, adjust the length of the straps so that the top of the ring is level with any location between your belly button and your pelvis. Once adjusted, place your feet directly under the rings. The rings should be hanging just in front of your thighs. Place your hands inside the rings and lean forward into a "decline" push-up position.

Even though you are leaning out on an incline, the muscles of the chest are pushing on a slight decline. We call this a decline push-up. This is the starting and finishing position for the ring roll out. With straight arms (keep a slight bend in the elbow to keep it unlocked) lean out as far as possible into your best Superman position. We teach clients to touch their biceps to their ears in order to encourage them to reach their full range of motion.

At this point, you are half way through one repetition. The midway point between the feet and the hands is the most vulnerable point for failure. This point is considered the center of the core. To support the proper posture (tail bone slightly up) the core must engage. You are now recruiting more muscular effort from your core than you would from completing any sit-up type exercise while protecting your back and improving your posture. To complete the movement, pull both straight arms back into the decline position. You should have your weight leaning on the rings the entire time. Do not unload (take your weight off) the rings. Now, you have successfully completed one repetition.

The fitness industry is filled with exercises, theories and equipment based upon building core strength. I have heard presenters at the last few continued education clinics I have attended say they hate the word "core" and are tired of talking about it. I think it's a misunderstood word is therefore overused. Core training should not mean how many sit-ups you can do or how much weight you can crunch on the ab machine. Core training, in my opinion, is teaching and obtaining the correct posture throughout each repetition, period.

The beauty of the OR is that no matter what exercises you do with them you are pretty much guaranteed to improve your core strength. Just like any other exercise, however, you can injure yourself while using them if you perform the exercises incorrectly. However, I do feel that the OR provide a great opportunity to improve core strength, posture and any other muscle group being recruited per the exercise you have selected. A good pair of rings cost around $100, but will last a lifetime if well maintained. The OR can be mounted in the garage, to a pull-up bar, or even in the backyard if you wish.

Do not be afraid to add some variety to your program design by incorporating some ring work into your workouts. It may be a little intimidating when you start; however, the more you practice and the stronger you get with them the more comfortable you will become. Core strength is very important (probably more important than any other muscle group) and should be trained appropriately on a daily basis. Your core supports your posture, and good posture leads to less injuries. Keep up the good work.

Dehydration: Low Water Intake Can Cause Back Pain

"Hey Water Boy, water sucks! Gatorade's better!" A world famous line from the blockbuster hit *The Water Boy* starring Adam Sandler. Well, maybe not an Emmy Award winning movie, but entertaining none the less. Adam Sandler plays a mild mannered 35 year old water boy who works for the local college athletic department. On a daily basis he is harassed by all of the football players, and one day he snaps when the quarterback spits into his water cooler. Bobby Booshay (Sandler) charges the quarterback and unleashes the fury on him thrusting his body through the air and spearing the cocky QB right between the numbers. What a classic scene; it's one for the ages.

Anyway, I was reminded of this movie while reading a new fitness book that I recently picked up. *Total Body Breakthrough* is a collection of health, fitness and nutrition secrets from some of the business's most successful and educated professionals. My two mentors, Alwyn and Racheal Cosgrove, each have chapters in this book. One chapter I want to discuss is called "Secrets to Staying on Track during Weight Loss" by Kim Chase. In this chapter, Kim lays out 26 tips for keeping on the straight and narrow when it comes to trying to change your body composition. Number 12 is subtitled "Lots of Water," and states that we need to take in about half hour body weight in ounces every day.

For example, I weigh 230 pounds (105 kilos) and should be taking in about 115 ounces of water each day. The average water bottle contains 16.9 fluid ounces of water. This means I should be drinking 6.8 (round it up to 7) bottles of water per day. The average person sleeps eight hours a day leaving 16 hours in which we have the opportunity to drink. This breaks down to a little under a half a bottle per hour. That's not so hard to do if you think about it in these terms.

Another way to accumulate the required hydration level is to add a zero to your current body weight in pounds. That is how many milliliters of water you should be drinking each day. In my case, I should be drinking 2,300 milliliters of water per day. This recommended liquid intake is for pure water alone. This should not include juice, milk or any other fluids (especially caffeinated drinks, as caffeine increases dehydration).

One major benefit to drinking this amount of water every day is the flushing of toxins from the system.

Another chapter entitled "A Fresh Nutrition Paradigm," by Jon Le Tocq states that "very few people are sufficiently hydrated to function properly on a basic level." Le Tocq goes on to discuss that water is what gives structure to the intervertebral discs found between the vertebra in the spine. Dehydration leads to smaller discs or 'cushions,' and can greatly increase the risk of lower back pain. Dehydration can also lead to a decrease in the stability of joint cartilage. This in turn increases the risk of rheumatoid arthritis and can drastically decrease the fitness enthusiasts "training life."

Some tips that we all know but sometimes forget:

- If your mouth is dry and you are thirsty, you are already dehydrated. Make sure you do not go into a workout thirsty, as you will not perform well due to being so dehydrated.
- If you feel "hungry" after recently eating, you are, more than likely, dehydrated. One of the symptoms of dehydration is a "hunger" sensation. Try drinking 12 to 16 ounces of water and wait five to 10 minutes to see if the "hunger" sensation subsides.
- You can injure of even kill yourself by ingesting too much water. Understand that hydration is good, but too much of anything is harmful. Stick to the suggested drinking amounts and your body should feel much better and perform well during workouts.
- The only problem with drinking more water is your body will have to get rid of it more often. You are going to have to use the restroom, often so plan ahead of time. There is nothing worse than getting into the middle of a 20 minute high intensity workout and suddenly feeling the "need to pee" sensation. This makes every jump, step up, and kettle bell swing dangerous; these kinds of pressure can cause accidents to happen! If you begin hydrating more than normal, your body will have to get used to this new level of water intake. Allow seven to 10 days

for your body to adjust, and your frequent trips to the restroom will return to normal.

If you found this information to be interesting and would like to learn more, please give this book a read. I think you will really enjoy it. No, I don't get any kick backs or funds for referring you. I am an education junkie and find this book to be a great combination of information from every realm of fitness and nutrition. Depending on who you talk to, you will hear that "correct nutrition" is anywhere from 70 to 95 percent of the effort to live healthy and decreasing body fat. Fitness is vital for boosting the metabolism and burning away those unwanted calories. Hydration is the link between the two, and should not be overlooked or undervalued.

Total Body Breakthrough

The world's leading experts reveal proven health, fitness and nutrition secrets to help you achieve the body you've always wanted but couldn't get until now. Copyright 2010.

Taking a Deeper Look:
Benefits of Weightlifting for the Baseball Player
(Published In the NSCA Performance Journal 2011 - Volume 10.2)

Weightlifting (the clean and jerk and the snatch) and variations of these exercises are explosive movements primarily utilized by power athletes (football, volleyball, baseball, or track and field sprints, jumps and throws) with the intent to improve athletic performance. High school, college, and professional athletes can work with loads near or at their one repetition maximum (1RM). This heavy load is required to optimize the athlete's ability to increase power production. However, this should not be done year round. This article will discuss why weightlifting is beneficial to an athlete's performance, and will be accompanied by a seasonal weightlifting program outline designed for in-season baseball athletes.

Weightlifting has many benefits for each type of athlete, including baseball players. These benefits include an improvement in the components of physical fitness and athleticism and a potential decrease in the risk of injury. Below are some of the specific benefits associated with weightlifting.

Neuromuscular adaption (learning to move the human body in pattern) is the most beneficial result from weightlifting for youth athletes (ages 12 to 18). Well organized training programs will teach the correct progressions for lifting weights, and youth athletes will benefit by learning human movement patterns. These patterns are the basic movements that every individual should be able to perform (i.e., squat, pull, and press). Athletes of all ages can improve their flexibility, reaction time, coordination, and balance while performing variations of the competitive clean and jerk or snatch lifts (3).

Muscular strength and **power output** go hand in hand. The load (weight) on the bar provides a slight overload to the muscle (2). The muscle will adapt to that overload during the training session and will repair itself during the next 24 to 48 hours following the workout.

During that recovery period, the protein in the muscles rebuild the fibers allowing for an increase in both strength and power (force times velocity) production during the next training session (1, 5). This load can be 15 pounds for a beginning lifter, or as much as 355 pounds for an advanced lifter.

Muscular endurance and **cardiovascular endurance** are both improved while participating in high volume weightlifting (1). Endurance athletes (runners, cyclists, swimmers, mountaineers, etc.) can dramatically improve their ability to contract their muscles repeatedly by lifting a moderate load. This load replicates the specific demands placed on the muscles while performing their sport.

Full range of motion (FROM) is a major emphasis in weightlifting. Moving lighter weight in a greater range of motion elongates muscles while they perform a muscular and explosive movement. The athlete can improve flexibility, strength, and power production through a full range of motion weightlifting program (4). Muscular imbalances can be corrected performing FROM lifts. These imbalances often result from repeatedly swinging the bat on one side or throwing with a dominant arm.

Weightlifting can additionally positively affect **body composition** as well. Lower loads, higher repetitions, and completing fewer sets (two to three sets with 90 seconds of recovery suggested between each set) have a high potential to decrease body fat and produce a low to moderate increase in both hypertrophy and strength. A higher load with fewer repetitions and completing more sets (four to five sets, 3 minutes of recovery suggested between each set) has a low to moderate effect on body fat and a higher potential to assist in hypertrophy, strength and power. The power athlete wants to take advantage of the high load and lower volume training philosophy during the times in the season in which the athlete needs to be most powerful (explosive).

Weightlifting can also **reduce an athlete's risk of injury.** Due to the increase in these areas described above, the chance of injury is dramatically decreased because the body is better conditioned overall.

Injuries most often occur when an individual places his or her body in an atypical position and applies pressure to an exposed joint, or overloads a muscle that has not been properly trained to handle that load. Weightlifting increases the capacity of every major joint in the human body. Listed in Table 1 is the number of injuries that occurred during 100 participation hours in school sports (5). Notice the lowest rate of injuries occur in weightlifting.

Table 1: Number of injuries per 100 participation hours in each school sport.

Soccer	6.20
Track and Field	0.57
Football	0.10
Gymnastics	0.044
Basketball	0.03
Weightlifting	**0.0035**

Weightlifting programs should not remain stagnant throughout any given year. Below are descriptions of when to properly apply weightlifting programs into training schedules of athletes currently competing:

Off-Season
When implemented correctly, a weightlifting program can benefit the baseball player year-round. But during the off-season, lifting extremely light loads (45 – 60% 1RM) and light volume (3x5 = 15 total volume) can help to efficiently deliver blood flow to fatigued or injured muscles. Pushing freshly oxygenated blood to working muscles assists in rebuilding the muscles as well as increases the muscles' flexibility.

Pre-Season
During the pre-season, the load the athlete lifts should increase (70 – 85% 1RM) and should be paired with moderate to high volume (5x4 = 20 total volume). This will increase the strength in various exercise

movements (i.e., back squat, bench press, and dead lift) as well as some power production in exercises (40-yard sprint time improvement or increased vertical jump).

In-Season:

The in-season phase emphasizes power production (85 – 100% 1RM) with a much lower total volume (3x2, and 2x1 = 8 total volume). The heavier the load becomes, the faster the athlete wants to move the bar. The strength gained during the pre-season will lay a foundation for power production development in season. As the in-season grows closer to championship games or the playoffs, the volume should stay the same and the load should shrink (75 – 85% 1RM). This reduction allows the athlete to maintain, if not slightly increase, power production risking injury prior to an important season capstone.

Post-Season:

What is important during the post-season is maintaining power, speed and strength, but also staying healthy. Moderate loads (65 – 80% 1RM) should be moved quickly. Volume can stay about the same (8 – 12 total repetitions under load) where, again, speed is emphasized and the risk of injury from fatigue is minimized as much as possible.

This article has provided information demonstrating how safe and beneficial weightlifting can be for competitive athletes at any level, and has specifically discussed lifting programs for baseball players training year-round. Proper instruction of progression, implementation and program design are vital to learning and performing the lifts correctly and safety.

References:

1. Brown, LE. *Strength Training: National Strength and Conditioning Association.* 113
2. Hedrick, A. "Weightlifting movements: Do the benefits outweigh the risks?" *Strength and Conditioning Journal* 30(6) 26-33, 2008.
3. Kutzer, B, and Theodor, H. *Weight training: Lift your way to a lifetime of health and fitness.* 1-1 through 1-7, 2002.
4. USA Weightlifting: *Club Coaches Manual.* 2002.
5. USA Weightlifting: *Sports Performance Coaching Manual.* 2003.

Taking a Deeper Look:
Social Facilitation and the Theory behind Fitness: Training In Groups.

The social facilitation theory was discovered by a man named Norman Tripplett in 1897 through a series of observations compiled on competitive cyclists. The cyclist would perform faster splits (time per lap) when racing against one another than when riding solo (time trial) (4). The riders would not only achieve faster lap times, but high top end speeds as well. To prove his theory, he devised an experiment involving a very simple task and a group of children. He asked the group of children to reel in a predetermined amount of fishing line as fast as possible. This test was performed by placing the children in pairs and by themselves. Their times were recorded, and proved that the children increased their performances in the presences of others.

Robert Zajonc's "drive theory" adds to Tripplett's social facilitation theory by designating a task to be simple or complex. A simple task (a skill that is mastered) that is performed with or in the presences of others results in a high performance. As the task becomes more complex (un-mastered), the performance with or in the presence of others decreases dramatically (4). To improve in performing a complex task, the participant must experience something called "neuromuscular adaptation." Neuromuscular adaptation is the period of time that it takes for an individual to learn a movement pattern (2). For example, a person learning the correct technique of the clean and jerk (Olympic lift) can physically perform each movement when it is broken down into simple movements. The act of performing them all in the correct order is the pattern that takes time to master. With practice, the steps required to perform the lift are learned separately.

The lift is now considered "slightly mastered". The movements are still a bit robotic; however, with more practice, they are smoothed out and strung together, at which point the skill is considered mastered. Neuromuscular adaptation has taken place, and the body can now perform the movement autonomously (without much thought). The complex task has become simple.

A counter theory to social facilitation is called "social loafing." Social loafing is when an individual produces less effort performing a task with others than he or she would have alone. This theory was the result of a study performed in 1974 by Alan Ingham at the University of Massachusetts (4). Ingham asked individuals to pull on a rope (tug a war) that was connected to a poundage machine. This machine would indicate how many pounds of force the test subject was producing when pulling on the rope. The individual was first tested alone, and then with two other subjects simultaneously pulling on the same rope. What the subject did not know was the other two were instructed to pretend like they were pulling. On average, the subject performed at 82% of his or her maximal effort when pulling with the other participants.

This lack of effort was due to the participant's knowledge that he was not pulling the rope alone. This caused participant to subconsciously rely on the other test subjects to pick up the slack. This mindset is created when individuals performing group-oriented tasks, feel less accountable and therefore worry less about what others may think of them. The tasks at hand and the environment in which the tasks are performed dictate which theory is to be implemented, social facilitation or social loafing.

Social facilitation will occur when individuals work together; they feel a slight pressure to perform well for the group and to keep up with their peers. For example, a group of six is asked to complete as many rounds as possible of twenty body weight squats, push-ups and kettle bell swings in that order for ten minutes (these individuals are being asked to work with their own equipment and at their own pace but still in the presences of others). Each person in the group will naturally work to his or her maximal effort to keep up with or outperform the others.

Social loafing will occur when multiple individuals are working to accomplish a common goal (3). For example, three people are asked to row as many meters as possible in ten minutes (these individuals will work together on the same piece of equipment). Each participant can only pull on the handle ten times in a row before they need to switch out with the next person. Ingham's study tells us that the effort put forth by each individual will be slightly less than if that person was asked to complete it on his own with his own piece of equipment. Each participant feels that the others will pick up the slack, which actually causes everyone to work below potential.

Social facilitation is the theory behind group training. Group training is such an efficient and effective practice that it is implemented in almost every field; medical school students, military personnel, kindergarten students, martial artists, chemotherapy patients, fire arms trainees, physical therapy clients, first aid/CPR trainees and personal training clients all train in groups (1). A certain pride and camaraderie is developed within these groups, as members hold each other accountable and support each other throughout every session.

A recent test, lasting just over a year, that involved 250 clients from a small fitness facility in southern California showed a success rate, for an individual training in a group to achieve their fitness goals, was 51 percent (3). Clients who trained one-on-one with their trainer experienced a three percent success rate. The group-training clients also reported they had a more pleasurable experience and frequented the facility more often. The research behind social facilitation supports a group-training environment however; the task must be mastered prior to an increase in performance based on the presences of others.

References:

1. Cosgrove, A. *Counting Reps to Counting Revenue.* 2010. Slides 16-17
2. Kutzer B, and Theodor H. *Weight Training: Lift your way to a lifetime of health & fitness.* 2002. Ch 1. Pages 1-7
3. Myers, D.G. *Social Physiology.* 2004. Pages 709-711
4. Weinberg, R. *Foundation of Sports and Exercise Psychology.* 2009. Pages 13, 85-85

Taking a Deeper Look:
Remember to Breathe: Utilizing the Valsalva Maneuver.

It has happened to all of us. You are struggling to achieve one more repetition of an exercise and your entire body tightens up. You hold your breath and drive with every last bit of energy you can muster. You achieve the lift and rack the weights, and then it hits you. You are light headed, the room starts to spin, and you begin to panic breathe as your fingers start to tingle. You have to sit down or hold on to a piece of equipment just to keep you from falling over.

After a few seconds, the dizziness subsides and your equilibrium returns. Your breathing turns from fast and shallow to slow and deep and you begin to feel normal again. You have just experienced symptoms of the 'Valsalva Maneuver' (VM). Research shows interesting results regarding the use of the VM in general fitness and sports performance program designs. This article will take you deep inside the research of the VM and provide you with instructions on how to apply this technique to your exercise routine and/or your sports performance safely and effectively.

Let's begin by breaking down how the VM occurs. The VM is the result of taking in a large amount of oxygen and then holding it in. This usually occurs when performing an exercise with a large amount of weight (80% of a one repetition maximum or more) or during an isometric contraction (the contraction of a muscle or a group of muscles without movement). An example of an exercise with isometric contraction is a plank or a wall sit. When a large amount of oxygen is taken in and held the Glottis, the opening between the vocal cords, it closes. Once the Glottis is , the diaphragm and abdominal muscles contract (see figure 1.) to produce a massive amount of intra-abdominal pressure (4).

Next, let's take a look at the VM's positive and negative effects on the human body. The Glottis has closed, and a massive amount of pressure has begun to build up beneath it. This pressure adds much needed support to the vertebral column (lower back) and is the primary reason for the VM. Olympic lifters, as seen on television during the Summer Olympics, utilize the VM more than any other athlete. The core strength of the abdominal wall acts as a weightlifting belt to breathe against producing an extremely solid foundation around the spin (3). The more solid the foundation, the more weight the athlete can lift. Although it clearly has benefits for the weightlifter, this pressure does bring with it some negative effects. The VM quickly increases blood pressure and in turn decreases oxygen flow to the brain, which can result in dizziness, loss of vision or fainting (3). We now know the Glottis closing produces massive pressure buildup, and as that pressure builds up, the amount of blood returning to the heart (venous return) to be re-oxygenated drastically reduces (4). This in turn diminishes the amount of oxygenated blood flow to the brain and muscles.

This is the primary cause of the dizziness, tingling in the fingers and the muscle fatigue (1). Oxygen flow to the muscles is much like gasoline to a car engine. Without a consistent flow of gasoline, the engine will not work as well and will eventually stop. Similarly, the muscles require oxygenated blood to continue to contract at a high rate; otherwise, they will stop functioning. This proves why breathing during each repetition of every exercise is extremely important.

A 'partial valsalva' (PV) should be implemented during general fitness training (less than 80% of the one repetition maximum). Every exercise has three phases of movement: the preparation phase, the acceleration phase, and the follow through phase (2). The preparation phase is the less difficult part of the exercise. This is when you should take a deep breath. The acceleration phase is the more difficult part of the exercise, and is when that breath should be blown out. The follow through phase occurs very quickly as a transition between the first two phases.

For example, when performing a body weight squat, the participant should breathe in as she descends down into the parallel squat or seated position (preparation phase). The participant then transitions and begins to push her body weight back to the standing position while breathing out (acceleration phase). The follow through phase occurs for a split second at the top of the squat prior to returning back down for another repetition. Generally speaking, you should breathe in during the easier part of the exercise and breathe out during the more difficult part. This technique will keep oxygenated blood flowing to your muscles, brain, and heart, allowing you to perform more repetitions.

In conclusion, the valsalva maneuver is a vital part of sports performance when an athlete is under a heavy load. However, for the general fitness enthusiast, the VM can be dangerous. Holding your breath during exercise is generally not advised, especially for older fitness participants, as this may create issues with high blood pressure (5). The partial valsalva is proven to be a safe and effective way to breathe during exercise for all ages. If you need assistance learning to perform the partial valsalva maneuver for your exercise routine or sports performance, please contact our Arden Hills wellness team to schedule an appointment.

References:

1. Findley, B.W. "Is the Valsalva Maneuver a Proper Breathing Technique?" *National Strength & Conditioning Association's Strength & Conditioning Journal*. 25.4: Pages 52-53, August 2003.
2. Floyd, R.T. Thompson, C.W. *Manual of Structural Kinesiology: Fifteenth Edition*. Pages 158-159. 2004.
3. Kutzer, B. Theodor, H. *Weight Training: Lift Your Way to a Lifetime of Health & Fitness*. Page 4. 2002.
4. Lombardi, G. *"The Impact of Valsalva Maneuver During Resistance Exercise."* National Strength & Conditioning Association's Strength & Conditioning Journal. 21.2: Pages 54-55, April 1999.
5. Staff. *National Strength & Conditioning Association's Strength Training*. Page 339. 2007.

Taking a Deeper Look:
The "Runners High" While Lifting Weights?

Maybe you have felt it before. You're out running, maybe three or four miles out, and you begin to feel a sensation that is hard to describe. Some say their feet and legs begin to tingle as both the mind and body become highly stimulated. It's a state of euphoria during which a runner may feel like he can go on for hours. It is called the "Runner's High." Though there is no scientific proof of this sensation, the majority of exercise enthusiast and professionals swears by it. As a personal trainer, I'm curious if this "high" has value. The more I hear about this state of mind, the more I ask myself, "What causes this feeling?" "What are the benefits to pushing the human body to this point?" "Can it be replicated by participating in other physical activities?" Please join me as I dive into the factors behind the Runner's High.

First, let's look at what might cause this reaction. Many fitness professionals believe in the Runner's High, but they do not know how to prove it exists. Most agree that the human body releases a chemical mixture of endorphins, the brain's naturally occurring opiates, which combine to make a mood altering reaction during exercise(4). Attempting to perform a spinal tap on an individual pre and post activity was not feasible. Researchers were able to perform tests on an athlete after activity, and found an increase of endorphins in the blood stream. However, these endorphins were a reaction to the bodies high stress level, which could not transfer endorphins to the brain (2).

In some cases, this reaction can stimulate an emotion which would otherwise not occur. For example, a female marathon runner finished her race, took one look a puppy, and began crying. She simply said that she could not help but get emotional; she couldn't control her reaction. Others are not sold on this idea. After pushing their bodies for a long period of time, they simply feel nauseated. When asked about her Runner's High, 5K runner Annie Hinkier replied, "I feel like throwing up." Whether it is a state of euphoria or a state of nausea, everyone agrees that there is a dramatic change in the chemical mixings of the human body post strenuous activity (2). This leads us to the question, "is this reaction healthy?"

Pushing your body to a state at which it begins to chemically change causes other more expected reactions, such as sweating, increased breathing and muscle soreness. In the long run (no pun intended), participating in a physical activity which pushes the body to work at 65 percent of its maximal capacity or higher for at least 20 minutes or more can produce dramatic health improvements (4). Following a healthy nutrition and exercise program can act as a cleansing experience for the body, as lead to the following improvements (1).

- Decreased risk of cancer, high blood pressure, heart disease, high cholesterol, diabetes and premature death.
- Reduced or maintained healthy body weight or body fat percentage.
- Increased bone density, joint stability and muscular growth.
- Reduced depression and anxiety levels, improved psychological well being, and enhanced work and sports performance.

Many benefits of starting an exercise program can take place almost immediately, and can improve your body's daily capabilities in as little as three weeks (4).

Good news for you non-runners out there: the effects of the Runner's High can also be replicated by participating in physical activities other than running. Exercising at 85% of your maximal heart rate for 10 minutes or more can replicate the same physical reactions associated with the Runner's High (4). Rowing, swimming, biking, jump roping, stair climbing, weight training, cross training and high intensity training programs designed and implemented correctly by a certified fitness professional can produce the same euphoric chemical reaction.

In conclusion, the Runner's High is a chemical reaction that takes place in the human brain during prolonged exercises at a moderate to high intensity (4). Whether or not this reaction is legitimate or is more of a placebo effect is undetermined by researchers. Either way, pushing your body's physical activity levels appropriately can only result in positive physical improvements, such as prolonged life, improved mental wellbeing, and reduced risk of disease. All in all, exercising could produce the sensation of feeling "high" without giving you the munchies.

References:

1. Department of Kinesiology and Health. *Healthy Benefits.* Georgia State University (www.gsu.edu/fit/benefits) 2007.
2. Kolata, G. *Yes, Running Can Make You High.* The New York Times (Fitness). March 27th, 2008.
3. NSCA Strength & Conditioning: *Hand Book.* 2009.
4. Willett, S. *The Runner's High:* Lehigh University (www.lehigh.edu/~dmd1/sarah.html) 2010.